ESSENTIALS

STUDY SKILLS

For Nursing, Health and Social Care

STUDY SKILLS

For Nursing, Health and Social Care

Edited by

MARJORIE GHISONI
and PEGGY MURPHY

Lantern

ISBN: 9781908625656

This book is an updated and revised version of *Essential Study Skills for Health and Social Care* edited by Marjorie Lloyd and Peggy Murphy, published in 2008 by Reflect Press Ltd (ISBN 9781906052140)

Lantern Publishing Ltd, The Old Hayloft, Vantage Business Park, Bloxham Rd, Banbury, OX16 9UX, UK
www.lanternpublishing.com

British Library Cataloguing in Publication Data
A catalogue record for this book is available from the British Library

The authors and publisher have made every attempt to ensure the content of this book is up to date and accurate. However, healthcare knowledge and information is changing all the time so the reader is advised to double-check any information in this text on drug usage, treatment procedures, the use of equipment, etc. to confirm that it complies with the latest safety recommendations, standards of practice and legislation, as well as local Trust policies and procedures. Students are advised to check with their tutor and/or practice supervisor before carrying out any of the procedures in this textbook.

Cover design by Andrew Magee Design Ltd
Cover image reproduced under licence from stock.adobe.com

Typesetting and production by Newgen Publishing UK Ltd, Stroud
Printed in the UK

Last digit is the print number: 10 9 8 7 6 5 4 3 2 1

Contents

About the authors

Marjorie Ghisoni is a Lecturer and course lead for mental health nursing at Bangor University in North Wales. Marjorie qualified as a nurse in 1996 with Bangor University and worked as a community psychiatric nurse for a few years before becoming a lecturer practitioner part-time then a full-time lecturer in 2003. After gaining her PhD in 2012, Marjorie believes that compassionate understanding of the needs of people in all walks of life is the main component of healthcare skills, education, development and practice. Marjorie is also a regular blogger on compassionate care: see https://drmarjorieghisoni.edublogs.org.

Peggy Murphy is a Lecturer in adult nursing at the University of Chester. She worked as a nurse in acute medicine and cardiothoracic intensive care. She became a lecturer in 2003 and has had an interest in working with students to support inclusive practice in nurse education. Peggy was awarded a National Teaching Fellowship by the Higher Education Academy in 2014 for her work on assessment and feedback and how this influences students' academic development. Peggy has published and presented her work nationally and internationally in the sphere of pedagogy.

Paul Jeorrett has been a professional librarian for nearly 40 years. He began his career at the Zoological Society of London and then at various academic libraries until recently retiring from Wrexham Glyndŵr University. During his career he has taught information skills to staff and students in many disciplines. Good presentation skills have always been a passion for him and he brings his experience as a conference speaker and singer to help students embrace their performing edge in whatever they are doing.

Liz Lefroy is a Senior Lecturer in Social Care at Wrexham Glyndŵr University. Her teaching and research interests centre on the involvement of those with expertise through the experiences of receiving health, social care and social work services. She has developed creative and innovative ways of ensuring that this knowledge is embedded in the curriculum for social work. More information can be found at https://outsidein2.wixsite.com/outsidein.

Jacqui Maung is a Subject Librarian for Health and Social Care at the University of Chester. She gained her MA in Information and Library Management at Manchester Metropolitan University in 2010 and has worked at University of Chester libraries over the last 13 years, most of this time working to support the Faculty of Health and Social Care. A large part of her role involves designing and delivering information literacy sessions for a wide range of undergraduate and postgraduate programmes in the Faculty. Jacqui has a professional interest in developing information literacy skills.

Craig Morley is a Learning Developer at the University of Manchester. He is an editor for the *Journal of Learning Development in Higher Education* and Chair of the North West Academic Libraries (NoWAL) Academic Skills Community of Practice. Craig gained his PhD in Ancient History at the University of Liverpool in 2015. He has published and presented research across different disciplines both nationally and internationally.

Seren Roberts is a Lecturer in Mental Health at the School of Health Sciences, Bangor University. Seren graduated and registered as a mental health nurse in 1996 and worked clinically in a variety of clinical settings. Following her PhD in 2003 Seren embarked on a long career in mental health research in which she undertook quantitative and qualitative research prior to taking up a lectureship in 2014. In addition to teaching healthcare students at undergraduate level, Seren also teaches at postgraduate level and regularly supervises Masters, PhD and Professional Doctorate students within the School of Health Sciences. Seren is an experienced literature reviewer and has published reviews in academic journals. For this edition, Seren has contributed a chapter on developing literature-reviewing skills, a key skill for any student studying a health-related subject.

Tracy Ross is a Senior Lecturer in Acute Adult Care at The University of Chester. Tracy has been a nurse for 34 years and her experiences include adult nursing in acute and primary care. She has worked in higher education for 18 years. Her publications include research methods and critical thinking. Tracy has carried research into caring and has won an RCN Nurse of the Year award in education for her contribution to caring in nurse education.

Helen Thomas is a Librarian at the University of Chester. She qualified as a professional librarian in 1999 and has created many taught information literacy sessions for a variety of undergraduate and postgraduate programmes of study for the Faculty of Health and Social Care in her role as Subject Librarian at the University of Chester. Helen has professional interests in developing user engagement and information literacy skills. Recently Helen has moved into a new role as Research and Repository Librarian at the University of Chester.

Ella Turner is a Learning Developer at the University of Chester and has direct responsibility for managing a team of academic literacies and maths specialists. Ella has worked in education for over 10 years in a variety of settings. She has worked as a tutor for lifelong learning within a local community setting and as a lecturer and personal tutor in two further education institutions, before moving into higher education as a Learning Developer in 2013. In addition to her BA (Hons) degree, MA and Diploma for Teaching in the Lifelong Learning Sector, Ella has achieved Fellowship of the Higher Education Academy in recognition of her teaching and learning support. She is currently studying for a Doctorate in Education and is a steering group member for the Association of Learning Development in Higher Education (ALDinHE). Ella was the first in her family to attend university and it is her personal journey as a student that has developed her passion for learning and teaching, enabling students to make sense of and get the most out of their HE experience.

Paul Verlander is a Senior Librarian at the University of Chester. Paul began his career in libraries in 2000 in the research library of the Health and Safety Executive, which he later went on to manage. Paul moved into higher education in 2007, during which time he has developed a keen interest in information literacy. He has presented at a number of conferences including LILAC (the annual Information Literacy Conference) and has had his work in skills development recognised as an exemplar of best practice by the national JISC project 'Learning Literacies in the Digital Age'.

Introduction

We seem to have forgotten that care and treatment is fundamentally delivered through human encounters, despite the advanced technologies that underpin the processes or procedures at hand.

Oelofsen (2016)

In health and social care you will experience many human encounters that will stay with you throughout your entire working life. These encounters will make you think about your practice and about how we all, as human beings, navigate our way through life. Many will make you think about your practice, reflect upon an event in practice, or develop your values and standards or your own practice. This personal development in our lives is what we now know as lifelong learning or how we navigate our lives. We are learning all the time, but to get the best out of this lifelong learning we need to be able to identify when it takes place and to demonstrate to our employers that we are reflecting and changing our practice or life course as we go along. In this book we have developed the themes of lifelong learning, resilience and employability to help you to do this and to help you recognise your skills as they are developing. We have also identified areas of practice or study where you can develop your lifelong learning skills. The following is a brief overview of how you can do this.

Developing study skills is a way to help you negotiate the challenges of further or higher education and beyond into your chosen career in health and social care. This book will help you develop lifelong learning skills for your professional career and help you gain the confidence to argue for good-quality care for the people you will be working with.

In health and social care we have a professional and personal responsibility to do no harm and to aim towards providing the highest standards of care for some of the most vulnerable people in society. People do not ask to get ill or become vulnerable and they can be very afraid of what will happen to them. As health and social care practitioners, we need to be confident in our practice so that people can be confident in us.

This book aims to help you develop your confidence in your ability to find information quickly, to scrutinise that information for its robustness and to apply that information when meeting the needs of vulnerable people. This may appear easy in practice, but in reality it takes years of study and experience together with a healthy dose of self-reflection for it to work.

During your studies you will access a myriad of information. Developing study skills will help you be able to make sense of all of this information and give you tools to develop your own mindset for lifelong learning. Reading this book does not require any prior knowledge of study skills but simply an open willingness to learn about yourself and about what other people have found to be helpful in their own studies. Therefore, we are all dependent on each other to share information and to use information in order to improve health and social care services.

The book has been designed to build your skills step by step and to help you to scaffold your learning to become independent learners in the future. The book is designed to enable you to engage with activities to develop your confidence as a student. Our aim is to develop you through interacting with this book to become more confident learners. Each chapter can also be read as a stand-alone resource to support your learning, but we have designed the book as a journey as you begin and continue to develop your lifelong learning skills.

The three themes that will be threaded through each of the chapters in this book – developing resilience, enhancing employability and learning for life – we feel are very important for personal development and growth in health and social care. In our experience these are major concerns for many students and this book aims to enable students to learn more effectively to improve their professional and personal lives.

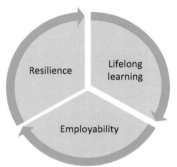

Developing resilience is interlinked with lifelong learning and employability as they each support one another. They are important factors for success in any chosen career, but it is through reflective practice that we become more aware of them. Reflective practice is discussed in more detail in *Chapter 9* as a tool to help us think about our individual resilience needs, what learning we need to do to develop our resilience and how will this help us to do our jobs well. We can also use the resilience cycle above to plan our future careers. Where would you like to be in 10 years' time and what knowledge, skills and experience will you need to be resilient enough to get there?

Developing resilience in health and social care

When we talk about resilience we mean the type of skills needed to flourish in an ever-changing environment such as education or professional practice. Having good resilience skills has been proven to improve self-esteem, develop self-confidence and, most important of all, demonstrate skills of compassion for ourselves and others.

Resilience requires a mindful approach to our everyday activities so that we can monitor our own responses. We will be asking you to do this in each chapter so that you can practise self-compassion and resilience skills. As you work through the book your skills will become useful in practice and in meeting educational and professional deadlines or requirements.

Developing resilience skills will also help you to identify your own needs when searching through literature and making reference to the literature that you have read. We will be exploring resilience as part of the learning outcomes in each of the following chapters so that you will become more aware of what skills you need to develop and increase your resilience skills.

Resilience is closely related to developing employability skills and lifelong learning skills, as without it we would be unaware of what our individual needs were. Therefore, developing skills in resilience will help you to do this as you learn about the human experience and all that it entails.

Learning for life in health and social care

Learning for life, or lifelong learning as it is more commonly known, helps us to develop skills that we can use throughout our career to update our knowledge and practice. As evidence-based practitioners this is really important and will help you to manage situations where people might say 'we have always done it this way' or 'why are we reinventing the wheel?'

Learning for life will add to your skills of resilience and employability as you will quickly be able to defend any decision you have made with up-to-date evidence or policy. You will find that learning for life is an essential part of your professional revalidation or continuous professional development portfolio. Whatever the reason you have for doing it, lifelong learning will help you to develop your skills of resilience and employability so that you can become a confident and compassionate practitioner. Most people with a desire to work in health and social care want to do so in order to help other people; however, as paid carers we need to know why we are doing things in more depth so that we can make sure we are helping and not hurting other people.

In each chapter there will be activities to help you to develop your lifelong learning in different areas of your practice. In a world where everything is becoming more demanding, it is important for our own resilience and employability that we are able to manage our individual lifelong learning needs and not become dependent on other people to do it for us. Lifelong learning is not a passive process but a creative, constructive and self-compassionate approach to personal development that can be of benefit to us and to the people we care for in both our personal and professional lives.

Employability in healthcare practice

Many students who enter health and social care courses do so in the hope of improving their job prospects and developing their career. They may have had many years' experience in the healthcare field but still feel as if they do not know enough to go for that dream job at the end of all their studying. If you bear in mind your employability needs and also those of your prospective employers, you can start tailoring your study towards your final goal.

For example, if you are interested in one area of practice you can focus your study in that area so that when you go for interview you are confident in your knowledge. You do need to be mindful of not being too narrow in your focus or you may find that you are very limited in the jobs that you can apply for. If you plan in the very early stages of your adult education or career how you are going to enhance your employability skills then you can gain the confidence in maintaining your knowledge base around the right areas of practice.

In an ever-changing world of health and social care we are as much influenced by law, risk and policy as we are by evidence-based practice. As professionals it is very important for us to get these sometimes conflicting views into perspective so that we can make sure we are practising safely and effectively. Sometimes conflicting views about practice can feel overwhelming so it is really important to develop our skills and confidence in our lifelong learning, employability and resilience. Most confident practitioners can utilise these skills and are able to demonstrate them every day.

If you can focus on these three areas you will be able to develop the knowledge and skills that make your personal and working life more fulfilling and beneficial to the people we want to help. To become a professional, however, takes more than just knowledge; it also requires an ability to self-reflect on and be mindful of what skills we need to improve and what skills we are quite good at already. We have made sure as editors that all chapter authors explore this in their chapters so that the knowledge and skills that you will develop from reading the chapter can be used to improve your employability. In a world where human encounters are at the centre of everything we do, the skills that we develop to deliver high-quality health and social care will be our toolbox for a long and satisfying career.

Conclusion

In this introductory chapter we have outlined how we think this book will be of most help to health and social care students. The activities within the book could also be useful to lecturers as ways of exploring practice and developing skills with students. We do hope that by taking a more general approach we are able to reach more students to develop and improve their skills in health and social care. In turn we are all aiming to achieve the same goal in that we can be confident that health and social care students are providing the best care possible to some of the most vulnerable people in society. Let us make it our aim as health and social care practitioners to develop the skills in lifelong learning, resilience and employability in every member of staff whose work involves high-quality and compassionate human encounters every day.

Marjorie Ghisoni and Peggy Murphy, editors

REFERENCE

Oelofsen, N. (2016) *Finding My Professional Heart: a brief guide to compassion and mindfulness for practitioners*. Lantern Publishing.

Chapter 1
Skills for the resilient learner

Peggy Murphy and Marjorie Ghisoni

LEARNING OUTCOMES

When you have completed this chapter you should be able to:

1.1   Develop your own resilience

1.2   Recognise skills of resilience in education and practice

1.3   Demonstrate awareness of resilience skills in everyday life and in the workplace

1.4   Apply knowledge of resilience skills to your lifelong learning and educational development.

1.1 Introduction

Resilience is identified by Windle (2012) as a measure of successful stress-coping ability or bouncing back in the face of adversity. When we talk about skills for the resilient learner, therefore, we are not just talking about skills that we develop to help us to learn, but also about skills that can help us to become a good person and consequently a good practitioner. As we all grow and develop we cannot help but become aware of the difficulties everyday life can present, from your computer breaking down the day before an assignment deadline to a sudden illness in your family. Resilience is needed to help us cope with everyday things just as much as we need it for our studies or working life. It is important, therefore, that we can start to recognise and develop skills for resilience in education, in the workplace for lifelong learning and in our everyday lives, so that we can become aware of how we can improve and develop them. This chapter will focus on developing skills in resilience in health and social care, but in each chapter that follows, we will also discuss resilience and how it can be developed in different areas of our educational and everyday lives.

1.2 Five ways (5Rs) to develop resilience for health and well-being

When we explore resilience in more detail throughout this chapter it will become evident that it is a process and that we all need to develop resilience in order to survive our busy working and personal lives. This is also known as self-compassion. Stress and depression are on the increase in higher education and in the workplace. If we ignore our individual needs to be more resilient then this might prevent us from developing the skills and knowledge that we need to find employment. The following five ways, or 5Rs, to resilience have been identified from many years of study by Ghisoni (2016) as ways to help us build our self-compassion as resilience skills. However, it is important to remember, as we perhaps focus on one way more than the other, that we are all global citizens with holistic needs and if we focus upon only one area of resilience, then it may not be as effective on its own.

1.2.1 Using REST to help us develop resilience

When we are under stress it is often experienced in different ways by different people, but it is important to recognise when we are stressed. One of the most common symptoms is not getting enough *rest* – for example, not being able to sleep properly because we are worried about meeting our deadlines. Sleep is a very important part of our resilience skills as it can also help us to improve our brain function and general well-being so that we can cope with stress better.

1.2.2 Using REPLENISHMENT to help us develop resilience

Another symptom might be not taking care of ourselves properly, which if unaddressed can lead to severe depression. It can be easy to forget to *replenish* our sleep and ignore hunger pains or eat the wrong food when we are trying to meet deadlines. It is important that you look after your body, because poor health can lead to lack of concentration and poor cognitive skills.

Griffey (2010) suggests that concentration is affected by a number of things including lack of food and lack of sleep. She argues, however, that it is better to have a good diet than to have a poor diet and take supplements. The brain is an amazing part of the body that is still being studied for information about how it works, but what we do know is that like any other organ in the body it needs to be well nourished to work properly.

1.2.3 Using REFLECTION to help us develop resilience

We have established that we need a well-nourished brain so that we can concentrate properly, but we also need it to help us *reflect* on what we do know and what we still need to know in order to increase our knowledge and skills. Reflection is important so that we can analyse our behaviour and the behaviour of others to see how effective it is in our practice as health and social care workers. Reflection, therefore, is the measurement of how we are doing and can be used every day. *Chapter 8* discusses how we can use reflective practice better to make us more resilient, but it is worth remembering that it is a very important part of our resilience skills.

1.2.4 Using RELAXATION to help us develop resilience

With all the hard cognitive work that we expect to be doing while studying, we also need to find time to *relax* and do the things we enjoy. The best way to unwind is some sort of gentle exercise like walking or swimming, but it can also be art or crafts. For example, there have been recent reports on how knitting is good for your mental health (Hickie and Randles, 2015). Anything that takes your mind off your studies will help you when you return to them so that you can concentrate better.

1.2.5 Practising RESPIRATION to develop resilience

Finally, the last point about resilience it is very important to breathe or *respire* properly. Many of us do not do this on a daily basis and it can lead to all sorts of health problems. If we consider breathing as another way of nourishing the brain cells then we will start to take it more seriously. Often this is due to bad posture or other physical restrictions, such as tight clothing. Griffey (2010) suggests that poor posture can also affect concentration by causing headaches, eye strain and muscular pain. It is therefore important to consider your desk space and chair to see how you can improve your posture and increase oxygen to the brain.

1.3 Developing resilience in everyday life

Developing resilience in our everyday lives is a good way to practise our resilience skills for other areas of our lives, including when we are studying for that next award or when we begin to work full-time in the increasingly busy world of health and social care. Therefore, it is helpful to think about how we might develop and practise resilience in our everyday lives.

Willis (2016) suggests that there are three ways in which we can develop resilience in our everyday lives quickly and keep developing it.

1. **Developing competence** – when we understand a complex problem we are also developing our competence and confidence in being able to fix the problem when it is broken down into more manageable parts. Writing an assignment can be daunting if we have not written one for a while. Breaking it down into manageable sections, perhaps using learning outcomes like we have done in this book, helps us all to cope better with a task.
2. **Learning from mistakes** – we can learn from something even when it has gone wrong, as we will have more information on how not to do it next time. Turning a negative thought into a positive thought will also help you to try again and not give up at the first hurdle. This can be done using skills of reflection, which we will talk about more in *Chapter 9*.
3. **Developing personal meaning** – thinking about how studying can help you, to improve care, for example, makes it much more meaningful to you. Here we can use stories and reflective practice to create deeper meaning out of our experiences so that we can learn more from them.

In addition, when we are helping other people to develop resilience, for example in the workplace or at home, we are also practising our own skills of resilience and making them stronger. Consider the following activity and reflect upon how you can help this person to become more resilient based on the three ways outlined above by Willis (2016).

ACTIVITY 1.1: HELPING OTHERS TO DEVELOP RESILIENCE

Omar was a student on your course who was having trouble accessing the online course material. He had been for countless tutorials with university staff but none of it was making sense. Omar was beginning to feel very disappointed with his poor grades and knew it was down to not being able to access the material he needed.

Reflective questions
How can you help Omar to develop his competency skills?
How can you help Omar to learn from his mistakes?
How can you help Omar to identify personal meaning in his experience?

HELPFUL HINT

There are some websites that have become very established at helping you to develop your resilience skills and they are worth visiting from time to time to help you to stay motivated when you are finding coping with everyday demands difficult. When you find one that you like, bookmark it on your computer so you can pop in and out for a break from your studies. Two popular ones are:

MindTools – A great site for helping you to develop skills around many areas of your working and home life www.mindtools.com

TED – Ideas worth spreading – as you can see from the title, this site shares ideas, but they are ideas from some very prominent people in the fields of business, science and education. Take a break by watching their short presentations online, which are always very professional and motivational www.ted.com

1.3.1 Using the internet to help develop resilience

It is tempting in this fast-moving world to have a quick chat with someone, sometimes a complete stranger, in an online forum, for example, rather than calling on people in your support network. This is becoming a common part of our everyday lives, but it is up to every individual to decide if this is actually helping them to develop resilience or not. Reflective practice as discussed in *Chapter 9* might help you to do this, but if you find that you are actually avoiding speaking to real people then chatting online may not be such a good idea. If you are concerned about how much time you are spending online, try keeping a diary for a week or two to see how you can change your lifestyle. You do not have to avoid online relationships altogether, but you may need to make them fit better with developing resilience in your everyday life, in your lifelong learning and in your employment.

Social media is also a great way to keep in touch with friends, and in health and social care there are many groups you can join on social media sites to discuss relevant topics. However, in all cases of using online support you must remember to follow professional guidelines for health and social care practitioners so that you do not break confidentiality. Your university website will offer links to helpful online sites and to places where you can learn safely – for example, Moodle or Blackboard.

HELPFUL HINT

Using online resources, which are often free, can be a great way to develop your resilience skills in everyday life, but always remember the following so that you use them safely and wisely:
1. Treat all online resources as public to remind you to think about whether you would say it in public or not
2. Do not give any personal details, especially bank details or passwords, as these can be used to hack into an account
3. Keep all of your passwords safe and try not to use the same one all of the time.

Many of the above suggestions for resilience in our everyday lives are transferable to our lifelong learning and employability skills in health and social care. However, we do need to think about these in a different way because the pressures and opportunities can be very different from our everyday lives.

1.4 Developing resilience for lifelong learning

Lifelong learning includes not only what we do in class or at home in our private study; it also involves taking a very broad approach to the learning needs of ourselves and others, locally and internationally. When you become a qualified practitioner you will be expected to attend conferences and visit other organisations or countries to broaden your knowledge base. However, as you develop in your practice you will also be expected to develop the service that you work within and to create new opportunities for people to improve their own health and well-being. In healthcare we call this Public Health or Health Promotion and you may be provided with the opportunity while you are a student to work or volunteer abroad to help people in developing countries to develop their own resilience. Lifelong learning therefore contributes to our Continuous Professional Development (CPD), which you will hear a lot about in the fields of health and social care.

Resilience in lifelong learning also means being able to identify what we need as individuals to develop our own resilience skills so that we can learn more about how to help others. In this section we will look at how resilience can help us to develop our lifelong learning skills. This includes looking for sources of resilience from within ourselves and from our local community network. This community approach is also known as global citizenship, which simply means that local people share resources to improve the resilience of the local or global community.

ACTIVITY 1.2

Consider what you would do to help people in your local community to develop their own resilience as a (global) community or organisation. Some real ideas are provided below.
- Making your local town a dementia-friendly town so that people with dementia can remain at home for longer
- Creating volunteering opportunities with local organisations for people with long-term conditions such as mental illness so that they can develop their employability skills
- Developing a healthy meals menu in a local nursing home to improve the physical health and resilience of older people
- Developing a community garden that produces food for local people.

You may have noticed that to set up these ideas you would need a lot of knowledge and skills around these areas of practice and that you would also need to make contact with other key people to help you. Therefore, when we are thinking about our CPD as practitioners, we are also thinking about what our lifelong learning needs are so that we can improve the lives of many people within our community. This is one of the major benefits of a global citizenship that can be an effective way of making the best use of local skills and knowledge, to develop resilient individuals and local communities.

The United Nations Educational, Scientific and Cultural Organization (UNESCO) recognises the role of education and lifelong learning in developing global citizenship:

> *In a globalized world with unresolved social, political, economic and environmental challenges, education that helps build peaceful and sustainable societies is essential. Education systems seldom fully integrate such transformative approaches, however. It is vital therefore to give a central place in Education 2030 to strengthening education's contribution to the fulfilment of human rights, peace and responsible citizenship from local to global levels, gender equality, sustainable development and health.*
>
> UNESCO, 2015, p. v

Global citizenship as outlined in the quote above suggests that in order to develop and grow our skills and knowledge we need to be able to see the bigger picture. In health and social care this implies being more holistic in our approach to practice. It is often difficult, however, to train ourselves to think in this way, and if you have not been asked to do it as part of your coursework it is worth keeping in mind that although people are complex beings we can consider three areas of their lives that could affect their development.

1.4.1 A holistic approach to lifelong learning

The following headings briefly outline how three basic building blocks can make us more holistic in our learning and in our practice.

Psychological – how we think about our skills and knowledge, and how we develop our thinking

Sociological – how we use our support networks to help us manage our daily life

Physical – how we take care of our physical needs so that we can continue with our studies

As we develop in our professional fields we might find that we forget about one or two of the three areas of holistic practice, but it is important to keep them in mind when writing assignments, or when taking care of ourselves so that we can get the best out of our learning. Identifying our own resilience skills can help us to identify other people's resilience skills. This is often what we call compassionate care, but it is very difficult to be compassionate towards others if we cannot be compassionate towards ourselves (Ghisoni, 2016). The 5Rs outlined earlier will help you to develop more self-compassion so that you are more able to help others do the same. The following scenario looks at how someone might develop resilience skills for themselves so that they can focus more on their studying.

ACTIVITY 1.3: TAKING A HOLISTIC APPROACH TO LIFELONG LEARNING

Jimmy is a young man who has left home to go to university. He was used to his mum taking care of him at home so is finding it difficult on his own. He house shares with two female housemates but he does not want to tell them how he feels. His coursework is beginning to suffer as he cannot concentrate any more.

Consider the following questions that Jimmy might ask himself. If you were Jimmy, how would you use the 5Rs to answer these questions?
Am I eating enough good-quality food to feed my brain?
Am I drinking enough to stay hydrated?
Am I getting enough sleep?
Am I worrying too much about my coursework?
Have I got enough support around me and do I need to make more friends?
Am I doing things that I enjoy to relax?

Thinking about global citizenship helps us to look at the wider picture so that we are not only developing our own knowledge and skills through lifelong learning but we can also help other people to do the same. This is a transformative approach to education that has been shown to help people learn by constantly applying what they have learned to themselves and to their place in the local community. As global citizens we are also more aware of the needs of others who might also have diverse needs. The above daily activities outlined for Jimmy could be increased if we start to add spirituality and resilience to the above list. It is important, therefore, to be aware not only of our own needs for lifelong learning, but of other people's needs too. This helps us to become more holistic practitioners and learners and will also help us to develop resilient lifelong learning skills that are compassionate for others and also compassionate for ourselves (Ghisoni, 2016).

HELPFUL HINT

Keeping a diary might help you to map your everyday activities so that you can identify where you might be having problems and might need to change. For example, if you spend too much time socialising you might not have any time left for studying.

1.5 Developing resilience for employability

In *Chapter 12* we will discuss resilience and employability in more detail, but it is important here to recognise why we need resilience skills to improve our employability as well as to develop our lifelong learning skills. Resilience in employability will help us to identify problems early and work out ways to address them. As the student Jimmy above had to look at his lifelong learning skills, we also need to do this for our workplace skills. In most workplaces our employers expect us to meet with them at least once a year to discuss our employability needs so that we can do our jobs well. Developing resilience skills by using some of the techniques outlined in previous sections of this chapter will help us to prepare for this meeting, which is often called a Professional Development Review (PDR).

It is important to see the term resilience in a positive way. Sometimes it can be used as a way of blaming people for not doing their job properly or as an easy and pat antidote to

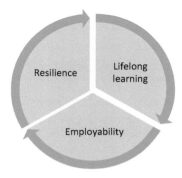

Figure 1.1 *The resilience cycle.*

the stresses and strains of busy working lives. Often these stresses are beyond our control, and this can lead to feelings of helplessness and even depression. This has consequences for both ourselves and our employers, as people become unable to work and need time off sick to recuperate.

While we cannot be certain that resilience for employability will eliminate stress in the workplace as targets and outcomes become a priority, it will help us to cope with the stress better. In this way we can see resilience as being a form of self-compassion where we learn to identify our own needs better (Ghisoni, 2016). This in turn will help us to be more compassionate towards other people as we become increasingly aware of our individual needs to do our job well.

Remember the five ways (5Rs) to develop resilience that we discussed earlier in this chapter. *Table 1.1* outlines how we can develop resilience skills in the three areas we have discussed in this chapter.

Table 1.1 *A holistic approach to resilience using the 5Rs*

Global citizenship	As health and social care students and employers we need to be aware of and reflect upon the needs of our local community to help us become more resilient.
	We also need to look at what affects people in our local community and prevents them from developing resilient lives – this includes the food that they eat (replenishment) and the air that they breathe (respiration).
	Finally, we need to look at opportunities to rest and relax in our local community and what resources are available, and utilise those resources.
Lifelong learning	As health and social care students we will need to develop our resilience skills and knowledge around rest and relaxation and how they can help us to improve our study skills. We will also need to develop resilience in our health behaviours and make sure we replenish our bodies with good food and respire properly to make sure enough oxygen is getting to our brains.
	We will also need to reflect upon our lifelong learning skills so that we can improve our employability and develop as holistic health and social care practitioners.

Table 1.1 *A holistic approach to resilience using the 5Rs* (cont'd)

Employability	As health and social care practitioners we will be expected to be able to reflect upon our lifelong learning needs and how we can address the needs of our employers. We will need to develop resilience skills so that we can do our work well, including making sure we get enough rest and relaxation, and replenish our bodies and respire properly to help us to rest, relax and repair our bodies.

The five ways of developing resilience take a holistic approach that can be applied in our everyday lives as well as in our employment and lifelong learning. Now complete the following table to identify how you can practise your resilience skills every day.

ACTIVITY 1.4: DEVELOPING PERSONAL, LEARNING AND WORKPLACE RESILIENCE SKILLS

Resilience skill	Employability	Lifelong learning	Everyday life	Notes to self
Rest			*e.g. always take lunch breaks*	*e.g. can be linked to relaxation*
Replenish				
Reflect		*e.g. always take notes*		
Relax	*e.g. go for a lunchtime walk*			
Respire			*e.g. practise breathing properly every day*	

1.6 Conclusion

Developing skills in resilience might be a personal way to develop your study skills in health and social care, but it is also very important for your individual success. In the following chapters in this book we will discuss how you can improve your skills in resilience in different areas of your studies. The most important thing to remember is to identify where you can get help and to access it. Resilience does not mean putting up with rules and regulations that make no sense to you. It is about making sure that you are aware of your own individual resiliency skills and that you know where and how to get the help that you need to develop them. In the fast-moving world of health and social care, being able to protect yourself in this way will demonstrate your valued contribution and integrity in any team or organisation.

In conclusion, there is no comprehensive guide to help you to navigate your way around every situation you encounter. You will make mistakes – we all do – so integrating resilience and reflective practice helps you to spend your time wisely. It is important to recognise when you have made errors and to learn from them. Do not waste time beating yourself up over being human.

Finally, remember that *you* have decided to study for a career in health and social care. Your journey will be challenging and rewarding and we wish you every success. In order for you to be successful in your course and career you need to invest time and apply yourself. If you are spending a lot of your time learning then it helps if you are determined to enjoy it.

SUMMARY

Five key points to take away from *Chapter 1*:
- ☑ There is no one way to develop individual skills in resilience.
- ☑ In developing your individual resilience skills it is important to think about your whole lifestyle.
- ☑ The 5Rs will help you to remember to Rest, Reflect, Relax, Replenish and Respire.
- ☑ Becoming a global citizen means helping local communities to be more resilient too.
- ☑ Developing skills in resilience will help you to enjoy and improve your studying more.

Quiz

1. What three things will help us to develop resilience in our everyday lives?
    a. Personal competence, personal meaning and learning from mistakes
    b. Personal meaning, personal understanding and personal skills
    c. Learning in practice, reflective practice, writing practice.

2. What does holistic practice mean?
    a. Psychological, cognitive and compassionate care
    b. Physiological, psychological and social care
    c. Spiritual, sociological and scientific care

3. What are the five ways to develop resilience outlined in this chapter?
    a. Reading, writing, reflecting, resting and reporting
    b. Reflecting, reasoning, resting, respiring and rewarding
    c. Resting, reflecting, replenishing, relaxing and respiring

4. What does Global Citizenship mean?
    a. Taking a holistic approach to developing resilience
    b. Taking a global approach to developing resilience
    c. Taking a personal approach to developing resilience

5. What does self-compassion mean?
    a. Only looking after yourself
    b. Being aware of your own needs
    c. Understanding your own needs

REFERENCES

Ghisoni, M. (2016) The components of compassion. Chapter 6 in Hewison, A. and Sawbridge, Y. (eds) *Compassion in Nursing: theory, evidence and practice*. Macmillan.

Griffey, H. (2010) *The Art of Concentration: enhance focus, reduce stress and achieve more*. Macmillan.

Hickie, I. and Randles, J. (2015) Knitting your way to a healthier, happier mind. The Conversation. Available at www.theconversation.com/knitting-your-way-to-a-healthier-happier-mind-46389 (accessed 30 August 2019).

UNESCO (2015) *Education 2030: Incheon Declaration and Framework for Action: towards inclusive and equitable quality education and lifelong learning for all*. United Nations.

Willis, J. (2016) The science of resilience: how to teach students to persevere. *The Guardian*. Available at www.theguardian.com/teacher-network/2016/jan/12/science-resilience-how-to-teach-students-persevere (accessed 30 August 2019).

Windle, G. (2012) The contribution of resilience to healthy ageing. *Perspectives in Public Health*, 132(4), 159–60.

Chapter 2
Effective time management
Peggy Murphy

LEARNING OUTCOMES

When you have completed this chapter you should be able to:

2.1   Consider yourself as an important resource

2.2   Manage your time effectively

2.3   Reflect on your current study habits to develop resilience.

2.1 Introduction

This chapter aims to guide you at the start of your journey towards your chosen profession and to support you in your lifelong learning. Embarking on a career that demands physical, emotional and cognitive labour is exciting and challenging. It can leave you feeling overwhelmed and exhausted at times. One way to help you maintain your health so you have sufficient energy to devote to your work is to manage your time effectively. None of us can pour from an empty cup. It is helpful to consider how to manage your time throughout the course, and throughout the rest of your career.

 IMPROVING RESILIENCE, LIFELONG LEARNING AND EMPLOYABILITY

Learning to manage your time effectively as a student will help you to develop resilience in managing your priorities when you enter the workforce. Good time management skills also contribute to your employability.

This chapter will help you to organise your time better through some interactive exercises. A key theme of this book is preparing you to sustain a career where you are constantly caring for others. In order to maintain this you must also invest some time and energy in taking care of yourself. Effective time management can help you to become more resilient because being a good time manager allows you to plan for rest and recuperation, and even recreation. Last-minute pressure can create a surge of adrenaline that helps to get work done over a short period of time, but if you over-rely on this technique you may find it comes at the expense of your health and well-being.

This chapter will help you to organise your time better to give yourself the best chance of success at university and life.

Transitioning into adult education after a more structured further education or A-level course can be difficult at first. You will be expected to take more control and complete a lot of work in your own time. Having to organise your own study may be new to you and you may need to spend some time developing a systematic approach to studying. Developing a routine can help you to get on with your work and prevent you from procrastinating. Many students complain that the two main problems preventing their progression on the course are:

1. Finding enough time to study, and then
2. Knowing how to use their time effectively.

Effective time management can help you to succeed. Each of us is allocated the same 24 hours in a day and 168 hours in a week. This same resource is available to everyone. Time is a 'non-renewable' resource: once it has gone, it is gone forever. It cannot be regained, or accumulated. Whatever way you decide to spend your time, you will still be allocated the same 168 hours per week as every other person. Some people have more commitments than others, but we all have things to do apart from study that take up time. Many students need to work to finance their studies, have families, caring responsibilities or may be part of a sports team.

Studying can place a great strain on existing relationships, because when you devote more of your time towards study, something else has to give in your life. All work and no play leads to a dull life. In order to maintain your well-being and your relationships it is important to allocate time to the things and people that you care about, as well as your study.

Getting the balance right can prove difficult, but it is important to avoid doing so much study that your health and relationships suffer. On the other hand, you need to allocate sufficient time to study otherwise you are unlikely to meet the demands of adult education. It is desirable to maintain a good work/life balance, to ensure success and happiness. Many students start off by overestimating their commitment to study, so it is important to be realistic about the time you are prepared to dedicate to your course in order to maximise your chances of achieving your goals. Setting unrealistic targets can undermine your confidence when you fail to meet your own exacting standards.

Effective time management can reduce your stress and improve your self-confidence (Payne and Whittaker, 2000). In order to develop resilience during the tough times, it is important to learn from mistakes and develop resilience and 'grit'. Duckworth (2016) argues that having passion and perseverance is important to success in life. She proposes that grit and determination are more important to success than natural talent. When planning your time, it is worth considering that it is both healthy and realistic to accept that you cannot do everything. It is also useful to recognise that you have choices in how you use your time, so ask yourself over the next day what do I have to do, what ought I to do, and what do I like doing?

ACTIVITY 2.1

Must do	Ought to do	Like doing

This activity is designed to help you to prioritise activities in your life. It can help you focus upon which areas of your life are important to you, such as relaxation, and which areas could *make way* for study time (particularly those that you found out you don't have to do). Some students write a daily to-do list using this 'must do, ought to do, like doing' principle to enable them to prioritise their day. Organising your activities reduces stress (Payne and Whittaker, 2000). During transitional times such as starting a new course at university, it is easy to allow key areas of your life to get out of balance; good time management skills help to focus your mind on giving sufficient time to meet the essentials such as family life.

Following *Activity 2.1* there are a number of revision questions for you to answer in *Activity 2.2*. These are designed to help you to refine your time management skills.

ACTIVITY 2.2

Ask yourself:
Q1 Why did I decide to start this course?
Q2 Am I making this time as enjoyable as possible for myself?
Q3 Can I do something to make this more enjoyable/interesting for me?
Q4 Am I taking things step by step?
Q5 Are my goals realistic?
Q6 How do I plan to reward myself for meeting my goals?
Q7 Do I eat/sleep/take breaks and relax enough?
Q8 Do I select certain aspects of my study to develop and leave others for another day?
Q9 Do I have an appropriate work area?
Q10 When studying, do I make myself comfortable?
Q11 Where I study is there enough light/ventilation?
Q12 Do I have all of the equipment that I need?
Q13 Am I likely to be interrupted during my allocated study time?
Q14 What time of day am I most productive?
Q15 What is the best time for new/more difficult activities?
Q16 Do I prioritise tasks before completion?
Q17 Do I postpone my studies? (First I need to … sort out my sock drawer/paint my nails.)
Q18 Am I aware of my weak points such as making a 'quick' phone call, or checking social media?
Q19 Do I take any steps to prevent distractions?
Q20 Could I use distractions more creatively? For example, if a friend calls could I ask them to take my kids out to the park for an hour?

2.2 **Strategies to combat time-wasters**

It is important to spend time recharging your batteries, as stated in *Chapter 1*. Rest helps you become more resilient. It is also important to recognise when 'rest' is turning into stalling your studies and preventing you from learning.

2.2.1 Internal time-wasting

Procrastination – everyone is tempted to put off tasks that are boring or difficult.
- **Possible solutions:** set deadlines and stick to them, use prompts so you do not forget, use a reward system when you have completed the task. If the task is overwhelming, break it down into bite-sized chunks to make it more manageable.

Perfectionist tendencies – do you waste time trying to get one element of the project perfect while the other parts suffer?
- **Possible solutions:** don't try to get it just right – just get it written! Remember most essays are written in several drafts before submission. Make a start then rework it.

Poor self-discipline – after committing yourself to study it does not always follow that you are consistently motivated to do the work.
- **Possible solutions:** remember that it is often the thought of work rather than the work itself that is the problem. Set yourself short tasks (a maximum half-hour time allocation) and motivate yourself with treats, especially when you have managed to work when you did not feel like it.

Anxiety – many students feel overwhelmed at times by the amount of work they have to undertake.
- **Possible solutions:** talk to friends and family, if necessary contact your General Practitioner and remember there are well-being advisors and a counselling service at most universities. Talk to your personal tutor or a peer mentor/guide. There are many self-help activities available to help you through tough times. If your anxiety is not out of hand, it may be worth considering that your time would be better spent by applying yourself to the work, rather than wasting energy worrying. When you keep yourself busy, there is less time to worry.

Poor organization – if you are untidy and unable to find your things easily you will waste time before you begin studying. If you get easily distracted, you will also waste time.
- **Possible solutions:** tidy up every time you finish studying, round off by putting your things away. Keep your focus on one thing at a time. Finish one task before starting a new one.

Over-commitment – this happens when you find it difficult to say no.
- **Possible solutions:** think about fulfilling your needs as well as everyone else's. Visualise the long-term rewards of being able to say no. Picture yourself with a

successful career, a higher grade. If you are asked to go out when you have planned to study it may be worth informing friends that although you are too busy right now you can offer an alternative time to socialise such as the weekend.

Inability to prioritise – some students find it difficult to concentrate upon the important tasks and get distracted by trivial things.
  - **Possible solutions:** complete a weekly 'must do, ought to do, like doing' list.

2.2.2 External time-wasters

Mobile phone – turn the ring tone off/do not answer/put the answer machine on/let people know you will call them back/get someone else to answer and take a message.

Visitors – be polite but firm. Let visitors know what times are convenient for them to call.

Television or social media – allocate yourself screen time or set a viewing time each day. Do not have more screen time than you have allocated. If you 'break up' study time with this as a reward, make sure that once you have had your allocated slot you return to your studies.

Travelling – if you travel on public transport then take a book with you, or review your lecture notes so you do not waste time looking out of the window. Listen to lecture podcasts or CDs on your subject area in the car.

Socialising – enjoy your time at university but try not to overdo it; limit this to after 9 pm or choose a set night for going out each week.

Crises – some crises are beyond our control, others are self-generated through poor time management.

ACTIVITY 2.3

Think about your own self-inflicted time-wasters. What are your ideas to solve these problems?

ACTIVITY 2.4

What might happen if you implement those solutions?

ACTIVITY 2.5: WORKING BACKWARDS FROM DEADLINES

When planning how to study for assessments it can be useful to organise your time by working backwards from the final deadline.

	How long will it take?	Personal deadlines	How long it really took
Brainstorm/reflect and discuss with others/formulate a plan			
First tutorial			
Gather information			
Reading and digesting the information gathered			
Grouping and organising the information			
Selecting what to include/leave out			
Improving first draft			
Improving second draft			
Second tutorial			
Improving third draft			
Writing up references			
Writing the final draft			
Proofreading and editing the final draft			
First deadline			

HELPFUL HINT

Create a positive learning space in your home. If you do not have a desk or table to dedicate to your studies then use a shelf, cupboard or storage box to keep all of your equipment together. Try to maintain the space so it is inviting to return to.

2.3 Suggested study toolkit

- PC, laptop, tablet or smartphone
- Books from essential book list (bought or obtained from library)
- A4 lined punched paper
- A4 ring binders for each subject
- Plastic pockets
- Small folder for current work; use file dividers to separate contents by subjects
- Personalise a notebook to use as your reflective study journal
- Diary, dictionary and thesaurus, if you do not already have these on your phone
- Address book for references
- Time planner/wall chart
- Pens, pencils, eraser, coloured pencils, highlighters, stapler, scissors, felt tips and ruler
- Something to keep you on track and make you smile, such as a plant, photo, poster or saying.

2.4 Conclusion

Developing good time management skills can help you cope with the demands of your course. Like all students you will have hiccups on your path to becoming a health and social care professional. There are a number of other skills that add together to enable effective time management and the activities in this chapter are designed to help you maximise opportunities for using your time effectively. Once reflective practice becomes more integral to the way you work, you can avoid wasting time berating yourself over mistakes and use your time more effectively by creating plans so you learn from difficulties and mistakes. Examining how you currently spend your time and completing a self-assessment of any time-wasting habits you have can help you to identify where you can access time to complete your studies. All of the skills learned in effective time management help you to see yourself as an important resource within your working life and knowing how to manage your time can ultimately help you to provide an effective service throughout your working life.

SUMMARY

Five key points to take away from *Chapter 2*:
- ☑ Poor time management skills can cause students to become stressed and less resilient.
- ☑ Resilience skills will help you to reflect upon your own time management skills and improve them.
- ☑ Working backwards from deadlines can help you organise your time better.
- ☑ Good time management skills are something prospective employers will be looking for.
- ☑ Managing your time well means you will have more time to do other things you enjoy.

Quiz

1. Why are good time management skills important?
   a. For meeting my deadlines
   b. For developing skills in resilience, employability and lifelong learning
   c. For having more time to spend with my family and friends

2. How can time management skills improve my resilience?
   a. I will have more time to plan and to think about improving my work
   b. I will be more confident in my study skills and will pass my assignments
   c. I will be able to help others to do their work more

3. What do I need to do to manage my time better?
   a. Talk to other people about my assignment workload
   b. Ask my tutors to give me fewer assignments to do
   c. Work backwards from my deadlines to make sure I have enough time to study

4. How can I avoid wasting time?
   a. Improve my self-discipline so I can prioritise my work better
   b. Take regular breaks for my work using social media, etc.
   c. Talk to others and ask for help with learning

REFERENCES

Duckworth, A. (2016) *Grit: the power of passion and perseverance.* Vermilion.

Payne, E. and Whittaker, L. (2000) *Developing Essential Study Skills.* Pearson Education Ltd.

Chapter 3
Reading and note-taking skills

Marjorie Ghisoni

LEARNING OUTCOMES

When you have completed this chapter you should be able to:

3.1   Find appropriate information quickly and efficiently

3.2   Write clear and concise notes

3.3   Be able to plan a review of the literature

3.4   Understand how reading and note-taking skills will help your employability.

3.1 Finding the right information

This chapter will help you to develop your understanding of the different types of information available and will lay some foundations for skills you will develop in subsequent chapters.

One problem that students in higher education often have is the feeling of being overwhelmed by the amount of information that is available to them, and they often wonder where they should actually start looking. To begin with, and before you start looking for information for your assignment, you should spend some time thinking about what type of information you will need. This will differ for the different assignments that you are given, so do not be afraid initially to cast your net as wide as possible to help you explore the information available. Then you can begin to narrow it down to the most appropriate information that you will need. In *Chapter 4* you will explore these skills in more depth, but to develop your ideas you will need to start looking at the broad literature first.

Figure 3.1 provides an overview of the many forms of information that you may be thinking about but, for academic purposes, you will also need to be thinking about which types of information will provide you with the most accurate evidence for your assignment. The Quality Assurance Agency for Higher Education requires education establishments to demonstrate that you have achieved a level of learning by providing evidence for that level of learning (see *Chapter 5* for more information on levels of learning). Therefore, you will be expected to have explored beyond the everyday information that is available to

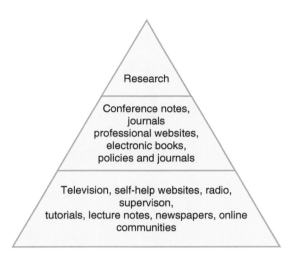

Figure 3.1 *Types of information available.*

all of society, such as that found in newspapers and websites, to other more challenging arguments for your ideas. While it may be useful to use quotations from the media to provide examples of what you will be studying, you will also need to explain why you have used a quotation and how this may influence your writing.

ACTIVITY 3.1: FINDING APPROPRIATE INFORMATION

Read the following and consider whether it would be suitable for an assignment. You may want to make a note of why you think it is or is not suitable for discussion with your tutor.

My brother's first joint and his descent into a mental war zone

The *Observer*, Sunday 13 January 2008, Alexander Linklater

In the summer of 2005, there was nothing particularly new about the onset of one of my brother's episodes. It was frustrating and sad, because Archie had at that point been doing well for some time and there is always the faint hope in manic depression that a remission might somehow take root and become permanent. But the symptoms were familiar enough: restlessness, the sudden announcement of grandiose plans, bouts of rage – and then the wild paroxysms of mood and personality that can lead to psychosis. Or madness, as Archie prefers to call it.

What was slightly different was the recent appearance of news reports on further studies into the links between cannabis and mental illness, with the emphasis on a genetic vulnerability to the drug. It was a subject that had gradually been worming its way into public consciousness, and my family felt the potential implications acutely.

The above exercise may help you to begin to plan how you will access information by following a certain lead or story and developing your assignment around it. There may also be other cues such as the assignment title – is it specific enough to tell you exactly where to start looking, or is it so vague it could mean anything? Your tutor will help you get started if you are having difficulties, but it is worth demonstrating that you have thought about the subject in advance of arranging a tutorial. You may also want to try out your mind-mapping skills, which are discussed in *Chapter 6*.

3.1.1 Search engines

Searching for information is covered in depth in *Chapter 4*, but we will look at some basics here.

Internet search engines are one of the most common methods that you will use to find information quickly. Unfortunately, some search engines return more accurate results than others and, if you do not define your search words adequately, you will discover thousands of links to your search. In addition, the information provided may not be of the standard required for you to develop your knowledge beyond common knowledge. For example, Google is the most popular search engine and there are many other less well-known sites, but you must remember that they are only search engines and they will find whatever you ask them to find, combining your search words with their algorithms. They will often return results that are irrelevant and omit the information that you really need.

3.1.2 Finding reliable evidence

Most search engines will not determine whether what they find for you is reliable evidence – you will have to do that. Google does provide a 'Scholar' site, which will tell you in the search whether it is a book, a paper or a citation elsewhere and the link will direct you to the source. However, unless you have online subscriptions to the many journals available, or an unlimited book budget, you will soon find your search resulting in a dead end. It is therefore important and very useful to you to become familiar with the online journals and library catalogue in your university so that you will immediately know you are searching reputable and available sources.

3.1.3 Using your university/college library to help you

You may also use the library facility to put a hold on books (from home) and access online study guides provided by your university. Wherever possible it is better to use your own university guides rather than those provided by another university. While you may prefer the layout belonging to another university, your own university guidelines will be based upon the assessment criteria that will be used to mark your work. Most universities will subscribe to online journal search engines and will subscribe to some or all of the journals in the search engine. Therefore, you will know that whatever you do find you will be able to access the whole article/book and not be prevented by a subscription fee or denied access altogether.

ACTIVITY 3.2: USING SEARCH ENGINES

Taking the time to hone these new skills on finding information that you need quickly is very important when you begin your course. You should not leave it until an assignment is due. You can practise this by typing some key words into one of your university's search engines and test yourself on the following points:

1. How did you refine your search from too many to a manageable amount of links?
2. How long did it take you to get one document/book?
3. Did you change anything to speed up the process and, if so, what did you do?

These will be useful discussion points for tutorial or peer support.

3.1.4 Finding information quickly

When you have discovered an article or book that you think may be useful to you, you will need to find out if it is worth locating, printing or downloading the whole article or part of the book (there are copyright laws that do not allow you to copy more than a certain amount of text from a book). You will therefore need to look at the overall document to see if it contains the information you need – this is called 'scanning'.

You can do this by reading abstracts and looking at the subheadings. You will also find that you can learn a great deal about what is in the book or article from the index and reference list and by looking for your keyword(s). Don't be convinced just by the title as these are often used to grab your attention and there are some interesting titles that have little or no relevance to what is actually in the paper. When you think that you have found what you are looking for you will have to speed-read and yet still obtain the information that you need to support your assignment. The three Ss below may help you to remember that in order to find information quickly you will need to:

- **scan** the document or book to
- **see** if it is actually what you are looking for and, if so, then
- **speed-read** the whole document to find the information you are looking for.

Speed-reading is an activity that students will develop in an ad-hoc way, but it can be organised to save the student a great deal of time. There are also free computer packages such as ReadPal available on the internet that will help you to skim through documents and some books on your computer screen. There are many books and apps on speed-reading now available that provide useful advice on how to prepare yourself to read through a large amount of material in a short time. Some of the hints and tips provided are quite obvious but worth remembering:

- Clear your space of anything that you will not be reading/using – it is amazing how this also helps you to clear your mind
- Make sure you have a quiet space and time slot in order to read with no distractions and work out what time of the day is best for you
- Playing music can help to relax you and block out background noise, but music with lyrics will distract you; the relaxing and mind-focusing effect of playing classical music can help calm pre-deadline anxiety
- Make sure you have some way of making notes to make best use of the time or you will forget what you have read; find out how you record information best – this might be online or written in a notebook. A5 notebooks are a good size to carry around too
- Take regular breaks to aid concentration, move around every 30 minutes or so and take a complete break every couple of hours.

IMPROVING RESILIENCE, LIFELONG LEARNING AND EMPLOYABILITY

You can use your regular breaks from reading as resilience breaks to practise your resilience skills, as outlined in *Chapter 1*.

In addition, it may be useful to vary the methods you use for gathering information, as reading can be difficult if you are tired from a hard day at work or studying. Podcasts are downloadable audio articles that often provide information from the literature and latest research, or you can listen to discussion broadcasts such as those from BBC Radio 4, for example. Alternatively, why not look for some webcasts or videocasts of news items and speeches. Some well-known authors (and lecturers) are also creating blogs, which are online journals or diaries used to record their current thinking that would be useful in supporting your information.

Try looking at the blogs from your university if these are available, or those on current health and social care journal websites such as the *Community Care* journal website. Finally, online social communities such as Facebook, Twitter, etc. are becoming a growing networking and group learning area, with some students finding their layout and informality a preferable place to the formal environment of the non-virtual classroom. The problem with this development in learning and finding information is that whereas students have developed this informal networking skill quickly with the easy availability of technology today, some tutors have not quite caught up. This means that there is currently a difference of opinion about what represents valid 'evidence' for your work, and this will be an issue that each university will address differently.

On the other hand, there is no doubt that e-learning has become a frequent mode of learning, and becoming more familiar with your university or college Virtual Learning Environment (VLE) will help you to develop study skills in this area.

3.2 Making concise notes

When students first begin higher education study they seem to need to write down every word that is said by a lecturer or every word that describes some concept in a book or journal. You will soon learn that, with the amount of studying required, this becomes impossible and you need to find a way of making more concise notes (Godfrey, 2014).

IMPROVING RESILIENCE, LIFELONG LEARNING AND EMPLOYABILITY

Developing the skill of note-taking early in your course will help you become resilient and adapt more quickly to college or university life.

This is a skill that is usually developed on an individual basis, but here are some useful approaches that will help you save time later.

- Always record the full reference so that you do not have to go looking for it later
- Try using or developing your own symbols or abbreviations, but make sure you have a note of what they mean in case you forget them
- Pick out keywords and use a diagram to join them up, a bit like a spider diagram – this is discussed in more detail in *Section 6.3.1*
- Record words that are not familiar to you as a reminder to go and find out what they mean
- If you are using quotations then always record the page number of the quote
- Organise your notes in some way so that it is easy to find them
- Try to write information in your own words as this can help you to avoid plagiarism (remember that you will still need to reference the idea as belonging to someone else)
- Keep a notebook and pen with you at all times – an A5 size notebook is not too big or too small to carry around
- Loose-leaf notepads are not ideal because pages can become detached and lost. If you do use a loose-leaf pad, it is a good idea to keep the pages in a ring-binder, organised by topic.

A good habit to acquire is that of making an annotated bibliography as you read your books or journals. An annotated bibliography helps you record concisely the main ideas within a text and, if it is written well, it can simply be transferred into your assignment with a linking sentence.

SCENARIO 3.1

An annotated bibliography entry:

Kitwood (1997) argues that people who suffer from dementia are neglected in that professionals only focus upon their medical needs rather than the whole person. Kitwood suggests that there are many ways of helping people with dementia and that they should be acknowledged as people with a disability that has social consequences as much as, if not more than, medical consequences. He suggests that staff should attempt to develop relationships with people who suffer from dementia in order to maintain their 'personhood', and warns that a lack of therapeutic relationships may result in social 'malignancy'.

Kitwood, T. (1997) *Dementia Reconsidered: the person comes first*. Open University Press.

Your annotated bibliography enables you to read the literature in more detail but, instead of taking copious notes, you will be taking from your reading what you think are the main points. This will save you time later when you start putting the assignment together because it will be a simple task of cutting and pasting your text into the assignment. This is also a useful skill to start working on for later in your programme when you may need to write a literature review. This can be an assignment on its own or a chapter within a larger assignment or dissertation.

Jones (2015) suggests that note-taking is a good practice to get into for writing notes in lectures and will help you to get the most out of the time that you spend sitting down listening to tutors talking at you in the front of the class. In a poll on Twitter in December 2018 I asked people how they learnt best. The results show that we learn best by *doing* more than *listening* or *reading* or *reflecting*, and so taking notes can be a *doing* activity that will help us to learn more.

ACTIVITY 3.3: WRITING AN ANNOTATED BIBLIOGRAPHY

Find a recent article or book that you have read and practise writing an annotated bibliography entry for it. Try to remember that this is not just a writing exercise but a useful skill that, when used with confidence, can save you time. Remember the following points when writing your bibliography entry:

- Keep your word limit to around 100 words
- Identify the main points, findings and/or arguments
- Record the whole reference and page numbers if using quotations.

3.3 Writing a literature review

As your programme of study develops, you are more likely to be asked to write a literature review. This will most often occur in the third year of a degree programme, but may also be begun in the second year or the final year of a diploma or foundation degree. As frightening as it may seem, a literature review is simply a collection of articles or books that contribute towards a body of evidence. In the main, this will consist of current research and policy documentation that will require some critical analysis (see *Chapter 5*). *Chapter 4* provides a more in-depth overview of reviewing the literature, but for this chapter we will outline the main requirements that you will need to think about when you are making notes.

SCENARIO 3.2

Sally was coming to the end of her second year of a foundation degree on childcare and had been asked to write a 3000-word literature review on poverty and childhood. Sally had never done this before and was not sure how to go about the task. She did not know what type of information she needed to look for or how to find it. From what you have read so far, what could you say to Sally to help her get started?

There are a number of issues to start thinking about when asked to review the literature on a current subject. The following list is a guide but, as your skills and confidence grow, you may want to add some more that are specific to your own needs. As well as developing your organisational and time management skills, a literature review also demands the ability to find information quickly (see *Chapter 4*) and apply critical thinking skills to what you have found (see *Chapter 5*).

3.3.1 Issues to consider when planning to carry out a literature review

- **Plan** – in order to find information for a literature review, as Sally has been requested to do, she must first make a plan or mind map (**see** *Chapter 6*).
- **Keywords** – from her plan, Sally will be able to pick out keywords that she will use to find more information.
- **Search** – to find more information on a subject, Sally will use a hand search through individual journals or books and/or use a search engine.
- **Note-taking** – Sally will need to make some record of what she has found, either as hand-written notes, as notes in a citation manager program, such as RefWorks or EndNote, or on a portable electronic device such as a laptop or hand-held computer.

In the above scenario, Sally might search using keywords such as 'poverty', 'children' and, perhaps, words relating to other areas that she may have read around, such as 'social class', 'education', 'health', 'parenting' and 'income'. The more words used in a search engine the wider the search will be. However, a search can also be made using a smaller combination of the same words, for example 'child', 'health' and 'income'. As you practise using keywords to search the literature, you will become more familiar with what works best and in what combination, but be warned: this activity does take time and patience. Often when students say that they cannot find anything they have either searched too widely or too narrowly and have to learn that searching the literature is a study skill.

As you begin to gather information and, invariably, documentation you will need to consider how you will file the information so that you can find it quickly later. A simple filing box may be all that is needed, but it is also worth getting into the habit of creating your annotated bibliographies. Alternatively you can do all this online using citation manager programs such as EndNote or RefWorks.

 IMPROVING RESILIENCE, LIFELONG LEARNING AND EMPLOYABILITY

As your career develops in the longer term, you may find that you need additional qualifications, or you may be asked to carry out a literature review to find evidence that supports a change in practice, for example. Therefore, reading the literature and making good notes is a lifelong learning skill and it will stand you in good stead if you hone the skill during your studies.

3.3.2 Finding the evidence

Evidence-based practice, as mentioned earlier, is about applying what you have read to your practice and, as a student, you also need to be able to write about it. This requires some of the skills mentioned above, together with skills discussed in other chapters (see *Chapter 5* on critical thinking and *Chapter 6* on essay writing and reports). Before you begin your own literature review, you may also want to explore in more detail the process of finding information to conduct a literature review, as this will help you become more familiar with what is required.

The following activity can be done on your own or with some fellow students, and it will help you to identify the differences between a research paper and a journal article or editorial.

ACTIVITY 3.4

Find a journal article from a professional journal in your area of practice. Without reading the content in too much detail, scan the whole document for headings. You will quickly be able to recognise an original research article if it has the following headings within it (these are also discussed in *Chapter 6* on writing a research report). If it does not have them then it is probably a theoretical or opinion article.

- Title
- Abstract
- Introduction and background information
- Literature review
- Methods of data collection and analysis
- Results
- Discussion
- Limitations
- Conclusion
- Acknowledgements.

 IMPROVING RESILIENCE, LIFELONG LEARNING AND EMPLOYABILITY

Literature searching as an employability skill

As qualified professionals we are expected to be able to justify everything we do with up-to-date literature. If you can demonstrate an ability to search the literature and find evidence for practice quickly and efficiently, you will be enhancing your employability.

When you think about how much information you receive from other people, from the media and via your hand-held devices, you will quickly find yourself in a state of information overload. Developing the skills of reading to find the right information, digesting and making notes of the most relevant aspects, and knowing where to look for the research or evidence you need will therefore save you a lot of time in practice (Godfrey, 2014). Critical analysis skills are discussed in more detail in *Chapter 5*, but it is worth remembering that even though you may have no intention of carrying out any research in the near future, you will still need to know what information informs your practice and how reliable it is.

Some dos and don'ts when exploring the literature on any health and social care topic are shown in *Table 3.1* that will help you to establish good habits early in your course or assignment writing (Jones, 2015).

Table 3.1 *Dos and don'ts when looking for evidence*

Do	Don't
DO look at professional journals for the evidence	DON'T start by searching the internet – you will be there forever and not get any writing done as you get distracted with other information
DO learn how to take notes quickly and efficiently	DON'T use charity websites – they may be very informative but that information is for the public, not for professionals who need solid evidence to support their practice
DO use your university or college library staff to help you	DON'T copy other people's work or cut and paste from the internet because plagiarism software will pick this up
DO seek support from your personal tutor or study skills centre in your college or university	DON'T use the same reference too often in your work as this will make it very descriptive and not analytical
DO start as early as you can on any assignment, as finding the right information can take longer than expected	DON'T leave it too late to look for the evidence for your assignment

 IMPROVING RESILIENCE, LIFELONG LEARNING AND EMPLOYABILITY

Social policy as evidence

Often we have to look beyond research for our evidence or we rely on social policy and/or law to tell us what the research evidence is saying. It is always worth exploring the literature around policy and law as it is what guides us in our practice and we need to be very familiar with it when applying for jobs. We can often find guidance and policy for our practice in health and social care on government-funded websites and it is good to become familiar with these sites early in your education and career so that you can update regularly. Below are the two main sites for health and social care.

National Institute for Health and Care Excellence (NICE): provide clinical and policy guidance on health and public health that can be downloaded for free – www.nice.org.uk

Social Care Institute for Excellence (SCIE, pronounced 'SKY'): provide guidance and policy on good practice in social care; they also offer some free training packages online – www.scie.org.uk

Social policy is therefore increasingly informing our practice in the form of guidance and law, but it is we as practitioners who will need to be able to analyse and convert policy into practice. Reading and writing skills are therefore an essential part of the practitioner's employability skills toolkit in order to capture the right information at the right time so that we can help people in practice quickly and effectively. This is the reason that you are studying this book right now so that you too can make a difference in someone's life. As Philpott (2018, p. 93) suggests in her book *Being A Nurse*:

> *Our patients are the primary reason that we have good days; knowing that we have helped someone and made a difference in their lives is the best feeling, and when we see the change that we are making, we feel like superheroes (which we are).*

3.4 **Conclusion**

Preparing to write your first assignment often fills the student with dread at the thought of getting it wrong or not being able to find any information. With some careful preparation from the beginning, you can quickly learn to develop your own learning style and skills that will enable you to produce work that will achieve good marks. It is important to remember to use all the resources available to you, including your tutor, as they are there to help, not hinder you, and you will also develop your own confidence in your academic ability. Learning good writing skills at this stage in your development will enable you to go on to write for publication when you feel more confident. Unfortunately, many postgraduates are unable to do this because they have not developed the skills or the confidence to do so.

SUMMARY

Four key points to take away from *Chapter 3*:
- ☑ Good note-taking can save you a lot of time in the long run.
- ☑ Learning how to take notes helps you to gather the right information.
- ☑ Searching the literature correctly can save you a lot of time.
- ☑ Social policy is an important part of your evidence.

Quiz

1. Which of the following can you use in an assignment?
   Newspaper articles
   Websites
   Television programmes
   Lecture notes
   Books
   Journals
   Radio programmes
   Tutorials
   Supervision notes
   Research
   Conference notes
   Professional forums

2. Name three online resources for sourcing different types of information.

3. Which of the following will you need when reading articles and/or books?
   More than one answer is possible.
   a. Enough space
   b. Pens and paper
   c. Enough time
   d. Playing songs by your favourite singer
   e. Making notes as you read

4. Why should you learn how to take notes? More than one answer is possible.
   a. To save time
   b. To copy other people's work
   c. To make sure you have referenced properly
   d. To develop your study skills

5. Writing an annotated bibliography helps you to:
   a. Make copious notes
   b. Record the main ideas within a text
   c. Create a long reference list

6. In order to carry out a literature review you will need to do what? More than one
   answer is possible.
   a. Make a plan
   b. Identify some keywords
   c. Develop a way of storing the information found
   d. Know everything about the subject

REFERENCES

Godfrey, J. (2014) *Reading and Making Notes*, 2nd edition. Palgrave Macmillan.

Jones, B. (2015) *Note Taking: 10 simple steps to effective note taking*. HRD Publishing.

Philpott, L. (2018) *Being a Nurse: a personal guide from graduation to revalidation*. Lantern Publishing.

Chapter 4
Skills for literature searching

Seren Roberts

LEARNING OUTCOMES

When you have completed this chapter you should be able to:

4.1   Distinguish between the different types of literature

4.2   Identify how and where to find relevant literature

4.3   Undertake your own literature searches in a systematic way.

4.1 Introduction

Gathering information is a skill we use in everyday life. Think about how you decided which university to attend or how you chose the mobile phone you have. Typically, we use multiple approaches to gather information to help us make such decisions. We might do a search online for information, looking at specifications and comparing organisations or products to generate a shortlist. We may want to see the organisation or product in person and therefore visit some universities on their open days or visit a shop to view the products of interest. We may even ask people we know for recommendations. In doing all this we are gathering intelligence (knowledge) on the thing we want to make a decision about – for example, which university to choose or which phone to buy.

SCENARIO 4.1

John was new to university but had worked in a variety of retail settings before choosing his career path. He was quite familiar with market research, where people are asked about products, but did not know how this was developed.

Customer feedback is very important in health and social care and what we provide as a service needs to be both cost-effective and efficient in how it is delivered, otherwise we would be wasting a lot of taxpayers' money.

John's lecturer advises him to visit a place where all the market research has been done for health and social care. The National Institute for Health and Care Excellence (NICE) and the Social Care Institute for Excellence (SCIE, pronounced 'SKY') regularly review current research and advice on the best approach to take when delivering services in health and social care. All information is free and guidance and tutorials are often available too.

National Institute for Health and Care Excellence (NICE) www.nice.org.uk

Social Care Institute for Excellence (SCIE) www.scie.org.uk

There are many websites that provide us with a vast amount of information, but it is important to remember in higher education that when you are asked to produce the evidence we usually mean research evidence. While policy should always be based on research as it is on the above two websites, you will need to develop lifelong skills in being able to identify research evidence from the rest. Many students use charity or self-help websites as evidence, and while this is very important information for the public it does not always state where their evidence has come from.

4.2 Starting your literature search

Searching literature is about gathering relevant information from different sources as we do for many of our daily decisions, applied to a specific academic context. That is, when it comes to writing your essay for your university degree programmes, you will need to find relevant academic information about the essay topic.

 IMPROVING RESILIENCE, LIFELONG LEARNING AND EMPLOYABILITY

As you develop your information-gathering skills for an academic purpose, these skills can also apply to your skills for daily living and employment as well as underpinning your lifelong learning. Knowing how to gather and weigh up information for decision-making is important in all aspects of our lives, including our working life.

Increasingly, healthcare professionals are expected to base their practice on sound evidence. Evidence to support healthcare practices largely comes in the form of research literature. As a student and healthcare practitioner, you will be expected to identify, interpret, weigh up and critically evaluate evidence to ensure your practice is up to date (Smith and Noble, 2016; Williamson and Whittaker, 2017). Thus, developing your literature reviewing skills is an essential aspect of your professional development and lifelong learning skills.

ACTIVITY 4.1

Think about a recent decision you made. Write down the strategies you used to inform this decision, e.g.
- Where did you get the information?
- How did you access this information?
- What was the most useful information source?
- Did some sources weigh more in your decision-making?
- Why?

Having reflected on a recent experience, you will note that gathering information is an essential aspect of our lives and the more skilled we are at searching for information, the better informed are our decisions. In an academic and professional context, we gather information and intelligence (knowledge) through evidence-based literature.

4.3 What is literature?

Literature is any form of written work or text. Published books, poetry, reports, newspaper articles, documents and flyers are all examples of literature. However, literature sources for reviews in an academic context should focus on more formal publications, such as published journal articles, textbooks, reports or guidance. Smith and Noble (2016, p. 2) state that

> *Literature reviews aim to answer focused questions to: inform professionals and patients of the best available evidence when making healthcare decisions; influence policy; and identify future research priorities.*

Literature reviewing is about thoroughly examining the literature that we find. Aveyard (2014, p. 2) identifies a literature review as

> *The comprehensive study and interpretation of literature that relates to a particular topic. When you undertake a literature review, you identify a research question and then seek to answer this question by searching for and analysing relevant literature using a systematic approach.*

In doing so, Aveyard (2014, p. 2) highlights that

> *A thorough search and analysis of the literature leads you to new insights that are only possible when all the literature is reviewed together and each piece of relevant information is seen in the context of other information. If you think of one piece of literature as one part of a jigsaw, then you can see how a review of the literature is like the whole completed jigsaw.*

In order to carry out a thorough review of the literature there are four key questions you need to ask in developing your literature search:

1. What do I want to know?
   First, you need to know what your question is. Taking the example above about purchasing a new phone, your question might be 'which is the best phone for me?'
2. Why do I need to know it?
   Using the same example, you would want to have a phone that is suited to your needs, that provides value for money and is affordable.
3. Where will I find the information I need?
   For the example above, you would seek out information from a number of sources. These might include experts in mobile phones found in phone shops; phone specifications on flyers, magazines, adverts or online; online reviews; advice from friends and family, and so forth.
4. Do I limit the information?
   Here you need to think about whether you need to place parameters on the information you seek. For the example of a phone purchase, you might consider whether you trust

the judgement of all friends and family or whether the opinions and views of certain people hold more weight in your assessment. You might also consider how valuable an online review from five years ago is for current technology. Reponses to this question will depend on what you want to know and what sources of information you use. Limiting the information may also help you to reduce information overload, which can be a problem now that we have access to so much information on the internet.

ACTIVITY 4.2

Think about these questions in relation to the following scenario. A relative asks you to help them bandage a burned area on the skin of their forearm.
- What do you want to know?
- Why do you need to know it?
- Where will you find the information you need?
- Do you limit the information you need?

In relation to this scenario, you would want to know how best to treat a small burn or whether a bandage is the best way to dress a burn. You would want to know this to make sure your relative has the best chance of healing as quickly as possible, to avoid making the burn worse and to minimise the chance of infections. The sources of information might include a local pharmacist or other healthcare professional, you may look online for information, or you may examine a leaflet in your first aid box. You would want to look at information sources that are up to date to ensure the recommended dressings are still available.

These principles of information gathering also apply to academic literature searching. In the same way that you might seek information about which is the best mobile phone for you, in an academic environment you would want to know what the best available information on your topic is. For academic purposes, most of the information we need comes from literature. We use literature as sources of evidence for our decision-making in healthcare practice.

IMPROVING RESILIENCE, LIFELONG LEARNING AND EMPLOYABILITY

Using the literature in this way and developing lifelong skills in literature searching increases our employability skills because we are able to cope with or become more resilient to the demands of professional life.

SCENARIO 4.2

When making decisions about what we need to be searching for, it is clear that we will all have different requirements, so it is important to make sure you are searching for the right types of literature.

As a new student, Sally wanted a phone that would:
- Be big enough to read documents on
- Allow her to access her university emails
- Download any apps she might need
- Keep in contact with her friends and family back home
- Make short notes on what she had read
- Take lots of photos of her time at university.

4.3.1 Types of literature

Deciding the types of literature you want to use is an important step. This will determine where and how you search for literature. In the example for *Activity 4.2*, you may wish to include information sources relevant to burns and grazes. However, you are unlikely to include information sources that relate to surgical wounds. This is because these wounds will require different dressings and you want to know the best type of dressing for a burn. Thus, you select some literature but exclude others to fine-tune the information that you are using for your decisions. While in the broadest sense your topic of interest is wound dressing, you are specifically interested in wound dressings for burns and grazes and thus wound dressing for surgical wounds would not help. It is important to select information as specific to your topic as possible. Applying selection criteria to your literature search enables you to use only relevant information for your decision, thereby ignoring information that is unhelpful to your decision. The selection criteria in the wound dressing example would be to include literature relating to wound dressings for burns and grazes (inclusion criteria) but exclude literature relating to surgical wounds.

ACTIVITY 4.3

Consider what types of information would be helpful for the two examples earlier of selecting a mobile phone and identifying the best wound dressing.
- Are the same types of literature needed in both examples?
- How might they differ?
- How might the questions you are asking guide the types of literature that would be useful?

As Aveyard (2014) suggested in the quotation earlier, asking the right question at the beginning will help you to find the relevant literature more quickly.

4.3.2 How and where will you find relevant literature?

Once the types of literature to be included have been decided, it is then necessary to determine where the relevant literature will likely be found. In the earlier example of choosing a mobile phone, it was suggested that a possible information source might include online for information or seeing the product in person. In an academic context, it would be important to identify appropriate information sources for the topic area and the assessment or essay criteria.

Examples of evidence sources

Evidence sources in an academic health-related context will include electronic journal databases such as:

Embase – which can be accessed via university login, www.embase.com/login
PubMed – US National Library of Medicine, www.ncbi.nlm.nih.gov/pubmed
CINAHL – the Cumulative Index to Nursing and Allied Health Literature, https://health.ebsco.com/products/the-cinahl-database
Ovid databases, www.ovid.com/site/catalog/databases/index.jsp

Other sources include:
Cochrane library, www.cochrane.org and Centre for Reviews and Dissemination, www.york.ac.uk/crd.

Students often use Google Scholar. While the selection algorithms for the online academic search tool are not clear, it is superior to a simple Google search.

Using reference lists

Another way to identify relevant material is through an explosion of references. This means looking at the literature that was cited by a key piece of literature you have identified. Each piece should have a reference list which may lead you to identify further relevant literature on your topic. Similarly, look at literature which cites the key piece of literature you have identified. This is likely to be relevant to the topic area in the broadest sense, but may also lead you to identify more contemporary literature relevant to your specific topic area.

HELPFUL HINT

Try getting familiar with some of the above search engines early in your studies because they will be easier to use when you need them for writing assignments.

Make sure you jot down any good references that you find.

Make a note of how to refine your search, e.g. years, keywords, etc.

Most academic journals are now available online with a search function. Thus, you can conduct an electronic search of specific journals relevant to your topic area. Taking the mobile phone example, if you had narrowed your choice to a specific make (e.g. Sony), then you may search the Sony website specifically. In the wound dressing example, you might specifically search the *Journal of Wound Care*.

4.3.3 Grey literature

Another source of literature for academic work is grey literature (Williamson and Whittaker, 2017). Grey literature is any

> *Information produced on all levels of government, academia, business and industry in electronic and print formats not controlled by commercial publishing i.e. where publishing is not the primary activity of the producing body.*

> ICGL Luxembourg definition, 1997

That means that any literature that is *not* a book or journal article will be considered grey literature. Examples of grey literature include: reports, discussion papers, theses and dissertations, newsletters, protocols and guidelines, Government documents (e.g. White papers), conference posters and presentations, etc.

Grey literature is not peer-reviewed (i.e. assessed by peers prior to publication to establish academic robustness, credibility and validity); this means the quality of the information might be variable, and the format of this type of literature can also vary. It is often produced rapidly, can be current and detailed, and is often free on the web. Conversely, some grey literature is costly to purchase or requires subscription fees, is not readily available through bookshops, can be intended for a small or specialised audience, may be geographically specific and on occasions is difficult to find. Topics which are not covered well in mainstream literature are generally found in grey literature.

ACTIVITY 4.4

Think about information you have used in previous academic work.
How would you classify the pieces of literature used for the information?
Were they research articles from journals or chapters from textbooks?
Were they from the grey literature in the form of government reports, newspaper articles or leaflets? Were all the sources appropriate to the information needed?

4.4 Developing a systematic approach to literature reviewing

We will now look at how you can systematically search the literature, developing your skills and knowledge as you go along. Like any skills this takes practice and you need to use it constantly to be able to confidently carry it out. The following steps will be discussed in more detail below, but are worth trying to remember or writing down in your notebook for when you start searching the literature.

1. Start by finding a *tool* you like and feel comfortable with – this can go into a table of all the literature that you find so that you can access it quickly when writing it up, e.g. PICO (patient/problem, intervention, comparison, outcome)
2. Use search *strings* to help you stay focused and on track, e.g. Boolean
3. Assess the *quality* of the research to see 'if it does what it says on the tin', e.g. CASP (Critical Appraisal Skills Programme)
4. *Analyse* your findings to develop a strong case (or not) for the service you are exploring
5. *Discuss* your findings using critical analysis skills with your peers and in your assign-ments. You can also make recommendations from your discussion which will inform your colleagues in practice and your tutors of your knowledge development.

These five steps, shown in *Figure 4.1*, should help you to find and explore the current literature, but please make sure it is up to date, as it cannot inform your practice if it is not. As tutors we usually advise that all research evidence should be within the last five years. These steps will now be discussed in more detail below.

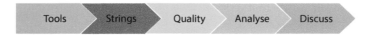

Figure 4.1 *A systematic literature review diagram of requirements.*

4.4.1 Developing a search strategy using tools

Once the topic area, literature types and databases are determined, the next step is to decide on the keywords or search terms you will need to use and how these are put together to build an appropriate search strategy for your work.

Importantly, your search terms need to be sensitive enough to capture as much relevant information as possible, but not so broad as to capture too much irrelevant material. Similarly, the search needs to be specific enough to mostly identify relevant material, but not too narrow that important literature is excluded. Getting the balance right between sensitivity and specificity can be tricky and may involve scoping the literature first by experimenting with the search terms to see what type of literature will likely be identified. This is why it is important to become familiar with the databases before you need them.

A commonly used framework for formulating search terms in healthcare is the PICO framework (Smith and Noble, 2016; Williamson and Whittaker, 2017), where
P is the population of interest (e.g. patients with burns)
I is the intervention of interest (e.g. wound dressing)
C is the comparator (e.g. alternative or no dressings) and
O is the outcome of interest (e.g. wound healing).

4.4.2 Using search strings

Building a search string (a list of search terms) using this framework helps to balance the specificity and sensitivity issues mentioned earlier. It is important to identify all possible terms relating to your topic (e.g. grazes, cuts, burns, wounds, etc.) and to combine them in a way that makes sense using the *Boolean* operators such as AND/OR, e.g. [Grazes OR Burns OR Wounds NOT Cuts OR Surgery] AND [Dressings OR Ointments OR Creams] AND [Healing OR Wounds). Use of medical subheadings terms can also help construct your search string. Depending on the nature of the review you are conducting, you may specify the study designs within your search string to identify only research literature of a specific type, e.g. surveys or wound care.

Once you have decided on the information you need, where you will find the information and the search terms you plan to use, your search strategy is complete. Following this systematic approach will ensure your literature search is relevant, comprehensive and replicable.

4.4.3 Assessing quality

The next important stage of a literature review is assessing the quality of a piece of literature that has been found (Williamson and Whittaker, 2017). You need to determine whether the information is useful, credible and trustworthy. That is, how much faith would you put in the information being provided? For this, you may consider the source of the information, the accuracy of the information, the robustness of the explanation (do you know how and why the authors have presented the information they have?) and what factors might influence how the information is presented and interpreted. For the mobile phone example, you might value the information provided by someone with personal experience of a given phone more than the company website. Why might this be the case? It may be that you suspect the company may publish biased information to help persuade you to select their particular phone. Thus, you might look at an independent review of the phone. This is also true for academic work. It is important to identify possible biases in the literature you review. For some reviews, acknowledging the possible bias is sufficient, but for others you may want to rule that piece of literature out.

There are formal processes for assessing and appraising the quality of the literature in healthcare, with many critical appraisal tools available. It is important to appraise literature to assess trustworthiness and relevance of information and findings provided. Developing your critical appraisal skills will enable you to make these judgements about the papers you identify. The CASP tools are a commonly used checklist in healthcare – see the website at www.casp-uk.net.

CASP considers research evidence in three steps:

Step 1: Assessing study validity – essentially, this stage is about evaluating methodological quality or the science of a piece of work to determine whether the study was biased or not.

Step 2: Considering the findings – if the work is deemed valid, then the next stage is to consider whether the information or findings are important to healthcare practice.

Step 3: Determining the value of the findings – if evidence is deemed to be valid and important, then the final stage is to determine how the information or findings relate to your question.

Critical appraisal skills provide a framework to clearly and explicitly consider these issues and will help you develop critical appraisal skills necessary for literature reviewing in healthcare. Developing skills to weigh up information and evidence for and against a practice, product and topic area is an important skill for lifelong learning and employability (Cottrell, 2017). Thinking critically about the information and literature you have sourced is a lifelong skill and is discussed in more detail in *Chapter 5*.

ACTIVITY 4.5

Thinking about information you have used for a recent decision you have made,
- How did you weigh up the information and evidence?
- Did some information hold more weight for the decision than the rest?
- How did you decide this?
- What factors contributed to you using the information or not in your decision?

4.4.4 Synthesising information and evidence

Once you have completed a search, selected, reviewed and appraised your literature, the next important step is to bring together the information and evidence into a coherent summary which highlights all the important points. There are a number of ways in which you can synthesise evidence (Williamson and Whittaker, 2017). For example, a *narrative summary* is a written description which tells the story of the evidence. A *thematic analysis* is about pulling out and organising the information from the literature into themes. A *meta-analysis* allows data from a variety of different studies to be pooled together for further analysis, while a *realist synthesis* aims to understand the complexity of interventions.

There are pros and cons to all the different methods for synthesising evidence. Some are better in relation to statistics, for example, and others are better for dealing with information pertaining to people's experience and views. The approach used for each literature review will depend on the question being asked of the literature, the types of literature to be used, the quality of the literature used and the similarity of the information and findings within the selected literature. Selecting the most appropriate and suitable approach to evidence synthesis is important and depends on the review purpose.

HELPFUL HINT

Go to your local library and look through the research methods books. These will discuss in more detail many of the issues around searching the evidence-based literature outlined above. Find one that you like and more importantly understand and either take it out on a long-term loan or ask your family to buy it for you as a gift. Becoming familiar with different research terms and literature will help you to understand what you are studying more as you become more able to critically analyse the literature. In particular pay attention to:
1. The glossary of terms – or make your own
2. Different types of research methodology
3. How to carry out a literature review (you may be required to do this later in your course)
4. How to summarise the literature (also see how to do an annotated bibliography in *Chapter 3*)

ACTIVITY 4.6

Thinking again about a recent decision:
- How would you present your case about your decision to your family members?
- How would you justify and rationalise your decision to them?
- What information and evidence would you present and how would you present it?
- How would you organise your information?

4.4.5 Discussing evidence-based literature with your peers

To help you develop resilience in this area of your skills it is often worth testing out your ideas with your friends and family. If you can explain your ideas or observations to them you can be quite confident that you can write your ideas down in an assignment. It is also useful to make use of tutorial time with your module tutors who may ask you to take part in a group tutorial or seminar. This is simply a way of sharing your ideas to make sure you are on track and not missing the main point of the evidence. It will also help you to develop arguments using the literature and avoid writing too descriptively, which often leads to poor marks in assignments.

In most professional fields, staff will get together over a lunchtime or after work to update their knowledge or continuous professional development (CPD) in a journal club, where they all discuss one research article. In the following example, a team of professionals might make the following observations from a recent policy that has been introduced to them.

SCENARIO 4.3: EXAMPLE OF A JOURNAL CLUB

Jo had just started working in a primary care GP surgery with many different professionals all in one base. Each patient is assessed by one of the staff who then helps them to address their individual needs. The staff are discussing a new local policy on blood tests. One of the doctors suggests that the policy is wrong because it is not evidence-based. Another asks why it needs to be. The doctor replies that they could be taking unnecessary blood tests if they are not needed. A nurse argues that this could cause distress as many people fear needles. A social worker suggests that this can then cause missed appointments and that there is research to suggest that GP surgeries waste a lot of time and money on missed appointments. The team agrees to look further into the evidence base for the policy before deciding to implement it.

The above scenario is common in professional practice as we are constantly under pressure to give a good-quality service that is evidence-based. Provision of good-quality services depends on individual people understanding and being able to apply the up-to-date evidence-based literature.

4.5 Conclusion

This chapter has highlighted the key concepts and steps for successful literature searching and reviewing. Information-gathering skills are essential in all aspects of our lives and can be applied systematically to searching for literature for an academic purpose. To do so effectively, it is important to understand what you need to know, why you need to know it, what type of information you need and where to find it, as well as how to select appropriate information. Choosing the right source material or literature will ensure your decisions are better informed and this is also true for academic work. The different types and sources of literature have been discussed, together with a description of how to construct a search strategy. Similarly, the ideas of assessing, appraising and synthesising literature have been considered. Continually developing skills in these areas, alongside your critical thinking skills, will not only ensure you have the necessary skills for successful literature searching and reviewing for an academic purpose, but will enhance your information-gathering skills for everyday life and decision-making. From this chapter you should now have an understanding of how developing literature searching and reviewing skills will support your lifelong learning and employability. Understanding these core ideas will enable you to develop your resilience when gathering information and knowledge throughout your life course.

SUMMARY

Four key points to take away from *Chapter 4*:

- ☑ Information gathering is an essential skill in all aspects of our lives.
- ☑ It is important to know what type of information you need.
- ☑ Assessing and synthesising the literature is an important study skill.
- ☑ Developing information-gathering skills will help you to make decisions in practice.

Quiz

1. Can you list three kinds of literature?

2. What are the key questions to ask when developing a literature search strategy?

3. What do we mean by inclusion and exclusion criteria?

4. What do we mean by assessing and appraising a piece of literature?

5. What does evidence synthesis mean?

REFERENCES

Aveyard, H. (2014) *Doing a Literature Review in Health and Social Care: a practical guide*. McGraw-Hill Education.

Cottrell, S. (2017) *Critical Thinking Skills*. Palgrave.

ICGL Luxembourg definition (1997) In Schöpfel, J. (2011) Towards a Prague Definition of Grey Literature. *Grey Journal*, 7(1), 5–18.

Smith, J. and Noble, H. (2016) Reviewing the literature. *Evidence-Based Nursing*, 19(1), 1–3.

Williamson, G. and Whittaker, A. (2017) *Succeeding in Literature Reviews and Research Project Plans for Nursing Students*, 3rd edition. SAGE.

Chapter 5
Skills for critical thinking

Tracy Ross

LEARNING OUTCOMES

When you have completed this chapter you should be able to:

5.1   Understand the process of critical thinking

5.2   Apply the techniques of critical thinking

5.3   Challenge the literature you read with a more open and questioning mind.

5.1 Introduction

The French philosopher Descartes (1596–1650) is famous for his words: 'I think, therefore I am'.

Descartes used this term to differentiate things that absolutely exist in the world from those that do not. However, perhaps he should have said 'I think, therefore I might be'. This, instead, acknowledges that thinking enables us to consider options, accept or reject these options and develop new options. Throughout life, humans are exposed to vast amounts of information. Not all of it is relevant to the way in which we live our lives, and if we acted upon all of the information that we take in, we would have no capacity for actual living. The human brain could be compared to a database in that the amount of data available is overwhelming; Halpern (2013) refers to this as 'creating a paralysis of analysis'. Making choices about how to select data is complex so we have mechanisms for filtering information in order to make it meaningful.

How do we do this? We think critically. On an everyday basis we are exposed to information, we question the worth of the information, we assess the relevance, we compare the information with additional information and we apply critical reasoning in order to make sense of it or we reject it. Basically, we draw together information from multiple sources and analyse it in order to inform our daily decision-making.

SCENARIO 5.1: EVERYDAY CRITICAL THINKING SKILLS

Imagine that you are going to book a holiday. Do you just book any holiday? Consider the process and steps that you would use and write them on a blank piece of paper. You would probably:

Read something about a holiday somewhere or have a discussion about a holiday or observe a holiday on TV, for example. This would be termed a *premise* or idea that motivates your thinking.

Next you *generate some ideas* or possibilities regarding the type of holiday that you desire; for example, would it be somewhere hot or cold? Abroad or in the United Kingdom? Self-catering or all-inclusive? Close to nightclubs, far away from nightclubs, cheap or expensive, two-star or five-star accommodation? These are the *inclusion and exclusion criteria.*

Then you would *investigate* the holidays that currently exist. You may access multiple sources such as websites, travel agents, TripAdvisor, newspapers and recommendations from friends.

You may then *evaluate* the options that exist by comparing and contrasting them against your inclusion and exclusion criteria.

Finally, you reach a *conclusion* based on the data and book the holiday.

We apply the same process to multiple contexts, for example when purchasing a car, when shopping at the supermarket, when applying for a new job, when moving house. We persistently contextualise data, make reasoned analysis and arrive at informed decisions. This form of reasoning is a central part of our resilience to everyday living and is practised without thinking about it. One would assume that it would be easy to harness this skill and transfer it into academia, yet critical thinking appears to be the student's greatest source of tension.

Attending university can be an anxiety-provoking experience for many students. Academic writing is stressful and academic failure is the worst outcome for a student. Feelings of diminished personal accomplishment can have serious consequences because poor academic achievement reduces motivation and promotes disengagement as a primary defence mechanism. Critical thinking is the key criterion to gaining high marks in academia, but humans do not think in this way every day; they are pattern-seeking, story-telling animals. These natural skills are incongruent with the more advanced critical processes required for academia and this results in work being labelled as descriptive. *Descriptive work leads to lower levels of achievement* and an increased level of internal anxiety.

Despite using critical thinking in many everyday contexts, it appears that the process of transferability is problematic. This may be explained by the labelling process; giving the process a name such as critical thinking implies that it is of a higher order than the thinking processes that are employed on an everyday basis. In fact, it is the same thinking but slowed down and practised on a deeper level. If we can make critical thinking more ordinary we can reduce the stress. *Students, you do not need to worry, you think critically every day so you can do it in an essay.* However, critical thinking is a craft and, like most crafts, it requires deliberate engagement, nurture and practice. It is a mistake to equate critical thinking with intellect, as two equally intelligent students may think in very different ways.

IMPROVING RESILIENCE, LIFELONG LEARNING AND EMPLOYABILITY

The intelligent student who applies intellect without critique may achieve the academic objectives, but the student who applies the technique of critiquing will achieve a deeper understanding of those objectives and through deep, sceptical enquiry will be better able to demonstrate that understanding in the real world of work as well as in academic essays.

5.2 What is critical thinking?

There are many definitions of critical thinking, most of which include terms such as synthesis, analysis, evaluation, scepticism, logic, questioning and clarifying. Chatfield (2018) describes critical thinking as analysing and critiquing information in order to apply a logical and informed approach to problem solving.

The term 'critic' comes from the Greek and means 'One who discerns or is in a position of disagreement'. To be in a position of disagreement carries negative connotations and implies that an unfavourable evaluation is given. The implication is that criticism is an opportunity for fault-finding rather than an opportunity to cultivate intellectual and personal growth. However, this is criticism, not critique. There are fundamental differences between the two.

Criticism involves one viewpoint that contains personal biases and opinions to the exclusion of others; it is subjective and self-focused. Criticism implies finality and closure, whereas critical thinking is an objective, positive endeavour that opens the mind and liberates the process of cognition. Critical thinking is the starting point of intellectual dialogue whereas criticism is the end of the conversation and does not allow for analysis of our practice or service delivery.

Criticism	Critique
Involves one viewpoint to the exclusion of others	Opens the mind and liberates cognition
Is subjective and contains biases	Is objective and positive
Is self-focused	Is outward-looking
Implies finality and the end of the conversation	Is the starting point of intellectual dialogue
Does not allow for analysis of practice and service delivery	Encourages analysis of practice and service delivery

Critical thinking is not describing. 'This essay is too descriptive' is a term over-used by academics and it is exasperating for students to receive. Description does exactly what it says on the tin; description describes events from one viewpoint with no support or rationale. Description fails to challenge or offer any alternative explanations. For example, have a look at the scenario below.

SCENARIO 5.2: DESCRIPTION

The author decided to develop a standardised pre-printed handover sheet, as the present method of handover has some problems. Staff were using individual pieces of paper or notebooks to take information in and the author felt that this was not ideal. The handover sheet was given to all staff to complete each day. The author then stored the handover sheets in a locked filing cabinet once they had been completed, to ensure confidentiality. Every member of staff was reminded to use the sheet and eventually it became good practice.

In this example, the writer tells the reader about a proposed change that she feels is important. However, the writer does not provide any supporting evidence to justify the need for change. She could have explored the rationale behind the current practice. The writer could have provided some further information regarding the implications of the current practice. She could then have added strength to her argument by complementing it with some current research studies that have explored the impact of the current practice. She could have debated some alternative options and considered the strengths and weaknesses of each option. She could have presented the staff's opinions statistically to the manager.

The critical thinker would question the current practice and seek explanations for the behaviour. They would investigate alternative measures, be sceptical of these options by looking in fine detail at the rationality and then appraise the evidence around the available options. This involves the willingness to examine information from multiple perspectives in order to establish logic and reason and come to trustworthy conclusions. Becoming a critical thinker is more than merely reading, it requires a willingness to be open-minded. The critical thinker has an enquiring mind and needs to see more than the presenting picture – as the thinker sees more, they will naturally offer more.

IMPROVING RESILIENCE, LIFELONG LEARNING AND EMPLOYABILITY

Critical thinking is an integral element of competence for both academic success and employability. For students it is concerned with consciously evaluating the worth of literature in order to appraise its relevance, and for practitioners it is concerned with investigating and analysing treatment options in order to provide optimal person-centred care.

While much of our everyday thinking is taken for granted or *tacit*, it may still be regarded as critical, as even tacit knowledge engages intellect and logic. However, critical thinking is conscious, judicious and investigative. Critical thinking is concerned with slowing down thought processes and thinking more than once about potential options and consequences. Critical thinking involves reading information, pausing for thought and then pulling the information apart and questioning the information in terms of its rationality and its robustness. Critical thinking is an objective evaluation about the quality of a piece of work, it identifies the overall premise or message within the work, evaluates the logic, questions the strength of the evidence, compares and contrasts the work with additional work and then comes to an informed judgement about the worth of the literature in order to either apply the findings, to solve problems or reject the work in favour of more favourable work.

ACTIVITY 5.1: TYPES OF THINKING

Read the following fictitious scenarios and decide which one may be considered as *tacit* thinking, *criticising* and *critical* thinking.

1. Claire is a new student nurse who is attending the Accident and Emergency unit for the first day of her placement. She looks very nervous and is obviously unprepared for this placement. She is just standing about watching everyone while they are getting equipment ready for the patients to arrive. She is going to be a problem for a very busy unit as she lacks knowledge and isn't interested in the job.
2. Accident and Emergency Units are very busy places. The pace of work is fast and the work-force are very highly skilled professionals. Students attending placements on these units can be overwhelmed by the pace and the level of knowledge that is required to function competently.
3. Research by X (2018) explored the experiences of seven student nurses who had placements in Accident and Emergency units. Their findings revealed that student nurses felt high levels of internal stress and felt overwhelmed by the fast pace and the technological nature of the environment. On the one hand it could be argued that lack of preparation prior to the placement could explain the high levels of stress endured by student nurses, because the preparation for placements tends to be of a generic nature rather than specific to the clinical placement. This is supported by additional research provided by Y (2018), who interviewed a small cohort of student nurses in London who expressed that their preparation lacked infor-mation about what to expect on their first day of placement. However, the research was car-ried out on a small sample of five student nurses in one city. In order to be more reliable, the study could have compared the views of a larger cohort of student nurses and could have included nurses from multiple cities. Although X and Y are in agreement in that they have identified that student nurses encounter stress on their first day of placement in Accident and Emergency units, the reasons for the stress require more in-depth investigation with larger samples of students in multiple areas before any further recommendations for change can be made.

Answers

You should have identified the first scenario in *Activity 5.1* as *criticising* as it is very subjective and there are several inferences drawn without any supporting evidence.

The second scenario may be identified as *tacit* thinking as it describes the situation but does not investigate or add any supporting evidence. Furthermore, it lacks any questioning and does not make any comparisons.

The third scenario is *critical* for the following reasons. First, the work starts with a message that the author wants to convince you about and the author provides evidence to support the idea being presented. Secondly, the author then questions the idea and compares and contrasts the idea with additional information. Thirdly, the author identifies strengths and weaknesses within the work and suggests that in its current format the evidence is not strong enough to warrant making any changes to practice.

ACTIVITY 5.2: DEVELOPING CRITICAL THINKING

Access and listen to the video 'Welcome video from Tom' at https://study.sagepub.com criticalthinking and reflect upon how it can help you develop your critical thinking skills.

5.3 How to think critically: a six-stage process

There is no magic critical thinking pill that will enable students to mindfully engage with literature; however, there are processes that can help. There is no one standard model for critical thinking, but several authors have tried to provide useful frameworks, such as Price and Harrington (2016) and Chatfield (2018). The framework provided in this chapter consists of a six-stage process that can be used as a structure for critical thinking for both the academic and real-world working context.

5.3.1 Stage one: critical reading

The key to critical thinking and writing is critical reading. Close and copious reading is essential, as you cannot be critical in the absence of options from which to draw conclusions. In other words, how can you select options in the absence of variety? In practice, health and social care workers cannot enable clients/patients to make informed decisions if the practitioners are not aware of the strategies that exist. Critical reading requires the reader to focus intensely and engage with the text in order to question. Therefore, rigorous searching for literature is important. There are many sources of literature available to access, but not all of these sites will be academically credible or free from bias (see *Chapter 4* for more information on identifying relevant literature).

HELPFUL HINT

For the purpose of academic evidence, some search engines you should become more familiar with are:

Peer-reviewed professional journals and sites such as The Cochrane Library, www. cochranelibrary.com

Resources from professional bodies such as the Royal College of Nursing (RCN), www.rcn.org, and **National Institute for Health and Care Excellence** (NICE), www.nice.org

Credible, library-approved online databases such as CINAHL, Resource finder, International Bibliography for The Social Sciences (IBSS), Google Scholar

Social Care Institute for Excellence (SCIE), www.scie.org.uk

Political sources such as: The World Health Organization, Department of Health, Public Health, and National Government.

Books published by academically credible publishing houses.

To be considered up-to-date, book sources should usually have been published within the previous 10 years and journal sources within the last 5 years, although older sources are acceptable if they are relevant to providing background context or classic pieces of work. Many students make the mistake of accessing high-level texts that may be obscured by jargon, leading to students failing to engage with the literature. Students cannot question the content of literature if they do not understand what they are reading. It is important to access the level of literature that suits the individual student and then build on this as confidence develops.

ACTIVITY 5.3: ACCESSING APPROPRIATE LITERATURE

I recently had a first-year undergraduate student approach me for advice during a research class. The student stated they were struggling to understand the basics of qualitative research. I asked the student which literature they had accessed. The student replied that they had accessed Being and Time *by Heidegger. Although the book by Heidegger is a credible source for the subject area, it is very philosophical, with complex language and concepts that are considered high-level for first-year undergraduate students who are in their first semester of study. Instead, I directed the student to a more relevant level text that would enable the student to engage with the text.*

Critical reading requires an environment that is conducive to thinking, so it is important that students study at a time that suits their needs where they are unlikely to be disturbed, because the mind needs the opportunity to roam. For example, some people are what I would refer to as 'cockerels' who can study early in the morning, while some students may be 'night owls' who are more able to study late into the night. Everybody has their own personal inbuilt circadian cycle which determines their patterns for functioning; working against this natural cycle produces stress and dysfunction, so it seems plausible to work according to your personal cycle and according to your personal circumstances.

5.3.2 Stage two: identifying the premise

Authors can be compared to sales personnel in that each one is selling the reader their viewpoint or message. The uncritical reader is vulnerable to each sales person. Close reading allows the reader to focus attention on the author's message and to identify the key points within it. This involves separating the relevant data from the dross. This tends to be successfully achieved if the reader first reads the whole text in order to get a flavour of the work and then selects one paragraph at a time and consciously asks 'what is this author telling me?' Sometimes the premise is written at the beginning of the text, sometimes it is a sentence written at the end and sometimes it is a thread that is not explicitly stated but runs throughout the text.

ACTIVITY 5.4: TRY TO IDENTIFY THE AUTHOR'S PREMISE THROUGHOUT THE FOLLOWING SCENARIO

There has been a tremendous rise in the rate of uncaring practices over the last ten years within health and social care. This is evidenced in numerous high-profile reports such as Francis (2010), Keogh (2013) and Andrews (2014). All of these reports highlight deficits in providing adequate nutritional care, dignified care and safe care. In 2008 there were very few recorded incidents of unsafe practice, poorly nourished patients and lack of dignity shown to patients. One needs to question whether standards are slipping or whether reporting mechanisms are more robust now. Maybe the wrong people are being employed or maybe the nature of caring itself has changed and people expect something that workers are not able to provide? Research by Ross (2018) showed that nurses spend too much time completing paperwork and this impacts the extent to which they are able to enact caring behaviours. I would agree with this as I have seen this happen when I was a patient.

Which one of these is the author's premise?
1. We are employing the wrong type of people in health and social care.
2. There have been several reports written about lack of caring.
3. People are undernourished.
4. There has been a tremendous rise in the rate of uncaring practices over the last 10 years.
5. Reporting mechanisms are more robust now than 10 years ago.

In this example number four is the correct premise. The author wants the audience to believe that there has been a tremendous rise in the rate of uncaring practices over the last 10 years and all of the other information that is provided supports this premise. All of the other four options support the premise, as they contribute to the reasons for a rise in uncaring practices over the last 10 years. The next stage is to question the message and this involves being sceptical.

5.3.3 Stage three: scepticism

The most distinctive feature of a good critical thinker is the ability to be sceptical or open-minded. Being open-minded involves having a tolerance for new ideas and divergent views. Cottrell (2017) refers to this stage as holding polite doubt. This stage primarily involves questioning the extent to which the author's premise can be believed. The reader evaluates the extent to which the claims fit with known reality. The reader should ask:

- Do I believe this?
- If yes, why? If not, why not?
- How does this fit with what I currently know or understand about the issue, i.e. does it fit with the reality of practice?
- Is there any logic in the claims?
- Who else supports this premise; is there any additional support?

The reader is looking for rationality within the premise. They should then seek indications as to why the premise should or should not be believed, as outlined in the scenario above. Achieving this aim involves seeking out the various views and positions that exist regarding the issue under discussion and viewing the premise from as many sides as possible. This can be an unsettling process as often it calls for a period of reflection or internal inspection that encourages the reader to challenge long-held beliefs and values.

This could start with the reader asking:
- What do I currently consider to be true about health and social care workers?
- Are they motivated by caring attitudes?
- What do I see in practice?
- How does what I see support the premise?

At this stage the reader establishes a preliminary logic and either accepts or rejects the premise, but this is based upon only one form of understanding that is rooted in personal bias and experience. The reader now needs to look for support or refutation from additional sources in order to objectify the held beliefs. It is important to highlight that critical thinking is not necessarily concerned with seeking truth because one could question the extent to which absolute truths exist. Therefore, knowledge is not about what we know, but is concerned with what we believe we know. Two students can read the same piece of text and their interpretations of the text may differ, but that is not to assert that either is wrong. Common-sense understanding is impacted by socialisation, culture, exposure to the problems and self-awareness. Reality is merely a process of interpretation; hence, if one applies the method of critical thinking, the logic will be unique to each person. There are no right answers, just different ways of viewing things (Carroll, 2012).

Cottrell (2017) argues that scepticism is not about doubting everything because humans need to have some trust in the world to exist within it. Too much scepticism results in failure to commit to anything, while too little results in gullibility. Therefore, scepticism involves being selective about the number of messages to investigate because most assignments are constrained by word limits.

5.3.4 Stage four: arguments and evidence

The extent to which claims can be believed is impacted by the extent to which the author provides support for the premise. In order to be persuasive the author provides evidence as to why the premise should be believed. First, the reader debates the logic, and secondly they question the robustness of the evidence. If we return to the text in *Activity 5.3* we can see that several forms of evidence have been presented in an attempt to support the premise being made. Three separate reports are presented, one research study is discussed and the author also supports the premise with their own personal experience as a patient. Cottrell (2017) refers to these types of evidence as contributing arguments and states that they form the pillars of the argument. The more pillars, the stronger the support for the premise. However, not all evidence has the same academic credibility.

The hierarchy of evidence

Murad *et al*. (2016) advocate that a pyramid of evidence exists which places systematic reviews at the top and personal opinion at the very bottom (*Figure 5.1*). This hierarchy of evidence determines the type of evidence that should be used to inform clinical practice. Systematic reviews are placed at the top of the pyramid and are espoused to constitute the most robust form of evidence because they are regarded as objective, scientific, bias-free, repeatable and generalisable to the wider population. The pyramid implies that if the evidence is scientific, it is the best form of evidence to solve problems. This form of thinking is termed 'positivist or quantitative' evidence.

Towards the bottom of the hierarchy are cohort studies, case studies, reports and expert opinions, which may be considered qualitative or naturalistic forms of evidence. Clinical experience would also be categorised as qualitative. These forms of evidence are less scientific and have the capacity to be impacted by personal biases and small samples of

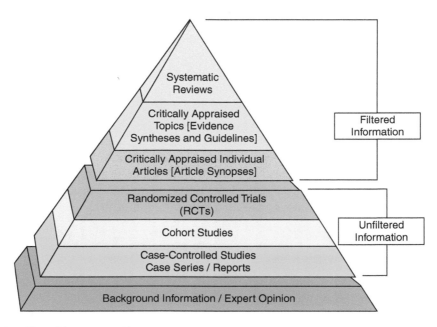

Figure 5.1 *The evidence pyramid.*

people. However, they have the capacity to provide rich, meaningful information, but it is not as generalisable to the wider population and so is not considered as relevant to the good of society as quantitative evidence. At the very bottom of the pyramid is opinion-based knowledge, which is considered anecdotal and too subjective for robust academic credibility.

The problem with this hierarchy is that it assumes that science can solve all problems. However, different problems require different solutions and science cannot adequately explain all facets of reality. For example, religious problems, cultural issues and the paranormal are rooted in belief systems rather than prediction and control. Furthermore, the human brain is complex and sometimes solutions occur on an intuitive level where the outcome is achieved without any logical explanation. However, despite its limitations, the pyramid does provide students with a starting point for evaluating the worth of evidence.

All forms of evidence have strengths and weaknesses and need to be evaluated for their rigour, which includes a consideration of the methods for acquiring data, procedures, ethics, analysis and theoretical consistency. This requires a basic understanding of research methods and the disposition to question. Several models exist to assist students with this process – Lobiondo-Wood and Haber (2018) and Ross (2012), for example. Most models contain similar criteria and include: evaluating the source of the work and where it fits within the hierarchy of evidence, the recency of the work, the compatibility between the theory and the methods, sampling procedures, ethical issues and approvals and analysis of the results. It is considered good practice to use the most up-to-date evidence, but this does not necessarily mean that a more recent study will be a more rigorous one, hence all criteria should be considered. Two additional issues should be included in a rigorous critique of evidence and these are reliability and validity. Reliability refers to the extent to which the findings can be replicated to achieve similar results, while validity concerns the extent to which the method or instrument used adequately represents the phenomena under investigation. However, the evidence is only as robust as the search performed, is only robust if it fits the problem at hand and is only as accurate as that which is available. Evidence is not fact, it is only evidence.

ACTIVITY 5.5: REFLECTING ON TYPES OF THINKING FOR LIFELONG LEARNING

Return to the scenario in *Activity 5.4* and identify the different types of evidence within it and consider where these fit in the pyramid of evidence.

5.3.5 Stage five: integrating the literature

This stage concerns drawing upon multiple sources of literature and debating them as a whole in order to strengthen your arguments. One piece of evidence may have many strengths and may add great support to your position, but there will be many that do not. The critical writer objectively compares and contrasts the variety of evidence that is available. Integrating literature is a very skilful task that improves with practice. In this stage the reader should identify commonalities and differences between the works and explain why they agree or differ. The student should also identify gaps in the knowledge and limitations in the work.

It is easy for students to commit two major sins in this stage, which may be viewed in terms of 'sunny day syndrome' and 'focus on the rain and forget the rainbow'. In the first, the student selects only those pieces of evidence that support their viewpoint and neglects those which do not. This results in the student offering a biased viewpoint and limits the extent to which they can be sceptical. In the second, students select all of the evidence but try to discredit the pieces that disagree with their viewpoint by highlighting the weaknesses and ignoring the strengths. This results in partial or flawed arguments.

5.3.6 Stage six: developing skills of reflection for lifelong learning

In this stage the student should reflect upon all of the arguments made and formulate informed conclusions. In *Chapter 8* this is discussed in more detail, but basically the student draws all of the information together in order to generate new thinking or theory. The new thinking may support the original premise or may cause the student to rethink their position. Reflection enables the student to consider the worth of what they are reading, but also motivates them to consider the robustness of their own viewpoints and this in turn produces a higher calibre of academic work. This reflective practice can then be practised in the work area to improve the quality of care delivered to patients and clients.

5.4 How does critical thinking improve resilience?

Benner (2012) argues that students suffer from stress because they care about the outcomes of their studies; she claims that caring sets up what matters and this in turn leads to stress and adverse coping.

Resilience is identified by Windle (2012) as a measure of successful stress-coping ability or bouncing back in the face of adversity. One of the key determinants of academic and professional resilience is critical thinking. Research by Kamali and Fahim (2011) found that good internal resources such as high levels of critical thinking ability and resilience can affect academic performance through enhanced reading ability and reduced levels of stress when students encountered the unknown, such as unknown words within complex literature. The deeper levels of thinking associated with critical evaluation led to an ability to cope with unfamiliar events. Kamali and Fahim (2011) found that critical thinking fostered higher levels of personal control, planning ability and comprehension. They also found that improvements in critical thinking were paralleled with improvements in resilience and vice versa.

5.5 How does critical thinking improve employability?

University education is not solely concerned with academic success. Universities have the wider objective of developing competent workers with higher-order thinking skills who can contribute to the stability of society. Critical thinking is therefore not just the concern of academia, it is a lifelong transferable skill.

From the work of Kamali and Fahim (2011), it seems reasonable to suggest that students who are able to reason critically, reflect and solve problems may be more resilient in the world of work as they are more able to problem-solve when faced with adversity. The application of critical thinking gives students the confidence to challenge events outside the academic context in a constructive manner. In practice placement and later in employment this includes challenging poor practice or creating opportunities for change. Halpern (2013) adds that the whole enterprise of learning would be of little value if the learning could only be used in the classroom.

Health and social care is rapidly changing. Workers face constant challenges and ambiguity and critical thinking is the antidote to habitual practice. Critical thinking drives health and social care forward; innovation can only be an outcome in a climate of thoughtful deliberation. Change has consequences and as such, it should be implemented on the basis of substantive and intellectual reasoning.

Modern health and social care is concerned with the nurture and care of vulnerable people. Therefore, health and social care professionals have an ethical responsibility to provide the highest level of person-centred care possible, based upon an assessment of individual need. In order to make informed judgements, health and social care professionals need to evaluate critically the range of therapies and solutions that are available and be selective. Health and social care requires decisions that are rooted in logical arguments and reliable evidence. Interventions need to be evaluated for their relevance, logic, safety and scientific merit. If health and social care professionals fail to critique the evidence that underpins their decisions they are doing vulnerable people a moral disservice.

5.6 **Conclusion**

This chapter has discussed the importance of critical thinking in academic life and proposed a six-stage model of critical thinking to direct students through the process. The first section defined the nature of critical thinking and identified it as a lifelong transferable skill that can be cultivated in the classroom, but this is not where it should stay. Students spend most of their lives in the world of work so academia needs to prepare students for the longevity of this and equip them with the most appropriate skills. Critical thinking is identified as a means of creating a more resilient workforce who are equipped to drive the future of health and social care. Resilience is a key feature of an empowered workforce who have the confidence to create innovation and challenge poor practice through the use of robust evidence and informed arguments. The six-stage model can be used as a framework for action in both academia and clinical practice, as being able to think critically in the midst of chaos is the hallmark of skilled professional behaviour.

SUMMARY

Four key points to take away from *Chapter 5*:
- ☑ Critical thinking can be carried out in six stages.
- ☑ Critical thinking prepares students for professional life.
- ☑ The six-stage model can be used as a framework for action.
- ☑ Critical thinking is the hallmark of professional life.

Quiz

1. What is understood by the term critical thinking?

2. What are the key features of critical thinking?

3. What are the six stages of critical thinking?

4. What are the benefits of critical thinking for students?

REFERENCES

Andrews, J. (2014) *Trusted to Care: an independent review of the Prince of Wales Hospital and Neath Port Talbot Hospital at Abertawe Bro Morgannwg University Health Board*. Welsh Government.

Benner, P. (2012) Educating nurses: a call for radical reform – how far have we come? *Journal of Nursing Education*, 51(4), 183–84.

Carroll, R.T. (2012) *Becoming a Critical Thinker*. Pearson Custom Publishing.

Chatfield, T. (2018) *Critical Thinking: your guide to effective argument, successful analysis and independent study*. SAGE.

Cottrell, S. (2017) *Critical Thinking Skills: developing effective analysis and argument*, 3rd edition. Palgrave Macmillan.

Francis, R. (2010) *Independent Inquiry into Care Provided by Mid-Staffordshire NHS Foundation Trust*: January 2005 – March 2009. Department of Health.

Halpern, D.F. (2013) *Thought and Knowledge: an introduction to critical thinking*, 5th edition. Psychology Press.

Kamali, Z. and Fahim, M. (2011) The relationship between critical thinking ability of Iranian EFL learners and their resilience level facing unfamiliar vocabulary items in reading. *Journal of Language Teaching and Research*, 2(1), 104–11.

Keogh, B. (2013) *Review into the Quality of Care and Treatment Provided by 14 Hospital Trusts in England: overview report*. NHS England.

Lobiondo-Wood, G. and Haber, J. (2018) *Nursing Research: methods and critical appraisal for evidence-based practice*, 9th edition. Elsevier.

Murad, H., Asi, N., Alsawas, M. and Alahdab, F. (2016) New evidence pyramid. *Evidence-Based Medicine*, 21(4), 125–27.

Price, B. and Harrington, A. (2016) *Critical Thinking and Writing for Nursing Students*, 3rd edition. SAGE.

Ross, T. (2012) *A Survival Guide for Health Research Methods*, McGraw-Hill, Open University Press.

Ross, T. (2018) *A Grounded Theory Study Exploring Nurses and Healthcare Consumers' Perceptions of Caring*, Unpublished Thesis. Glyndwr University.

Windle, G. (2012) The contribution of resilience to healthy ageing. *Perspectives in Public Health*, 132(4), 159–60.

Chapter 6
Writing essays and reports

Marjorie Ghisoni

LEARNING OUTCOMES

When you have completed this chapter you should be able to:

6.1   Plan the outline of an essay or report

6.2   Find information from a variety of reliable sources

6.3   Organise and compose an essay or report

6.4   Develop your knowledge of the essay writing process.

6.1 Introduction

It is not uncommon to feel nervous when you begin a course of study, with many unanswered questions running through your mind.

This chapter will help you answer some questions about how you can get the best out of your study time and enjoy the whole experience more.

 IMPROVING RESILIENCE, LIFELONG LEARNING AND EMPLOYABILITY

As you develop skills in writing essays and reports you will find that it becomes a lifelong learning skill that you will use in your everyday professional life and you will develop resilience around finding the right evidence to include.

Some colleagues talk fondly of their student days being the best part of their lives, and an enjoyable experience should be what you are also aiming for, not three years of anxious anticipation. This chapter will address some of the anxieties common to many students, such as:

■   How do I write an assignment, exam, essay or report?
■   What do I include?
■   What do I exclude?
■   How do I find information?

- How do I know if the information is good enough?
- And probably the most anxiety-provoking question – where do I begin?

This chapter will explore in more detail some of the skills you will need to develop in order to cope with the amount of work you are required to produce for your course of study. In addition, it will also provide you with an overview of the institutional requirements that guide most higher education courses. When your lecturers are preparing your courses and assessments, they are basing their requirements of your standard of achievement upon the standards required by these other professional bodies. This will be discussed in more detail later in this chapter but is acknowledged here to help you recognise the quality cycle that is in place around your academic study.

6.2 Begin at the beginning

Where to begin will depend upon what type of assessment you are expected to complete. There are many types of assessment such as written assignments, examinations, research reports, literature reviews, theoretical analysis, role-play and poster presentation, but for the purposes of this chapter, we will focus upon three main types – the written examination, report writing and the written assignment. All of these assessments, like most others, require a period of preparation and organisation.

You may also be asked to submit work for these assessments either formatively or summatively. Formative work, such as a mock exam or poster presentation, is informally assessed, while summative work is given a mark that is fixed and unchangeable. Formative work assignments are not always taken seriously because the student knows that they are not being given a final mark. However, formative work is a good way of obtaining feedback from which you can actually improve your final or summative mark, so it is important to know the difference and the value of each. Although formative work is more informal, the feedback may be more important and useful than in summative assessments.

Many tutors notice that students lack a systematic way of approaching their written work which, like any other activity, requires you to go through a series of steps to achieve a good outcome. For example, we learn to go through a number of steps to drive a car or it will not get us where we are trying to go. These steps become routine after a period of time, but to begin with, students may need a framework to help them. I developed the 'PROCESS Framework' of academic writing (Lloyd, 2007, p. 50) with those students in mind. The word 'process' in this context is an acronym for the steps or stages that are required to produce a robust piece of written work and they can be described as follows (*Table 6.1*).

All of these stages will be discussed in more detail below. The framework will also provide the student and their tutor with an outline of what needs to be discussed within tutorial sessions. This helps both the student and the tutor become better prepared to get the most out of the time available, as most often students are limited to a certain number of meetings with their tutor.

Table 6.1 *The PROCESS Framework (adapted from Lloyd, 2007)*

Planning	What is it you are trying to achieve?
Referencing	How will you find out what you need to know?
Organisation	How will you collect your information together?
Composition	What level of understanding is required?
Engineering	How will you construct your assignment?
Spelling	How will you know that you have the correct terms?
Structure	How will you present/argue your findings?

ACTIVITY 6.1

Think back to your last assignment tutorial and/or written feedback. Use the framework shown in *Table 6.1* to identify where you might have been able to improve your work and to identify what skills you may need to develop further.

6.3 **Make a plan**

Planning can be something you really do not think you have the time for, but it will be invaluable to help you keep on track while you are becoming organised. Planning helps you to map out your initial ideas, which you can then share with a friend or your tutor who can help you keep on track. The more elaborate your plan is now, the easier it will be to follow when you get nearer to your deadline. It is never too early to start planning. You will also need to think about how you are going to plan to deliver your assessment, which will improve the presentation when it is finished. These may seem simple suggestions now, but in the anxiety and confusion of a looming deadline they can help you to make sure you have remembered everything. For instance, have you thought about making sure you have all of the things in this list?

- The right equipment
- Enough paper, ink cartridges and pens
- Enough time to complete and print out the finished document
- Enough books and resources, or access to resources such as library/printing cards
- A quiet space for studying/reading/thinking
- A filing system for all the papers you will collect.

Some students create their own system of information storage, but this tends to happen later on in the course when they have learned from their past mistakes. One third-year student recently said to me, 'If only I'd known then what I know now', which of course is impossible, but their hindsight can be extremely useful to new students. Therefore, it may be helpful to use your peers as a support system, talk to them over coffee about how they plan and organise their study. Some universities have buddy systems where more experienced students support students who have just begun a programme of study. This is not the same as plagiarism where students copy other students' work, knowingly or not. The buddy system simply helps you to find your way around and become organised quickly.

ACTIVITY 6.2: MAKING A DEADLINE CHECKLIST

Start writing yourself a deadline checklist, which you can add to your calendar or diary well in advance of the hand-in date. Discuss with your tutor if you think you are going to have any problems. They may be able to help you access support. Above all, don't just hope that the problem will go away – it probably won't. (See *Chapter 2* for more information on time management skills.)

6.3.1 Mind-mapping

This activity can be carried out on a computer using specific programs, or on a piece of paper, whichever is more convenient for you to use. Whatever method you use, make sure you are comfortable using that particular method as you have no time for trying to find lost ideas when you start working on your assessment. This will only cause you further anxiety, which you do not need. You will have been given an assessment briefing, usually at the beginning of the module that you are currently studying, so will need to go back to the briefing to check what is required. There should at least be some learning outcomes like those at the beginning of this chapter, and maybe some further guidelines about presentation, etc.

A mind map (see *Figure 6.1*), also sometimes known as a spider diagram, is a collection of associated words on a page with linking lines and words to connect them all together. Mind maps usually begin with a central word or idea – perhaps the exam or essay title – in the middle of the page and then spread out in a sort of loose spider's web of related words and ideas – as many as you can think of. Once you can no longer think of ideas that might be useful to your study, you can move on to the next stage of gathering information on aspects that you now know you want to write about. Don't worry about forgetting something important as you can always add it later; for now, you have a plan that you can start working on.

As you can see from the basic diagram in *Figure 6.1*, finding information is not the only thing you have to think about when preparing for an assessment. However, finding the right information is more important than finding a large amount of useless information. When writing a report or exam your plan or mind map will help you to keep focused and prevent you becoming overwhelmed by the amount of information out there.

6.4 Referencing from journals and books

Some students are never quite clear whether they should be using journals or books for their information requirements. More frequently, students will use the internet to search

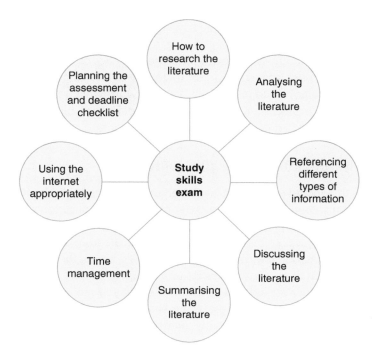

Figure 6.1 *Example of a mind map or spider diagram.*

for information, but this can lead them into more problems when referencing if they do not know how to do this properly. *Chapter 3* has provided you with the basic support needed to search resources successfully and, more often than not, you will have found yourself looking at a book or a journal article either online or in your library.

A student's preference for either books or journals becomes apparent when the submitted piece of work includes a reference list of only one or the other. This immediately informs the tutor that the student may be having problems when looking for information. As a basic rule, if your assignment is purely theoretical, books will usually be sufficient. However, if you are talking about practice, which you will be in health and social care, there also needs to be some evidence. Not many books simply provide evidence because their content is mainly the opinion of the author, whereas journal articles tend to provide the evidence in the form of research reports and analysis. A mixture of both books and journals in the references demonstrates an awareness of reliable information sources and the ability to apply them both.

Chapter 7 explains how to reference the information that you have found, but you should also remember that the way in which it is presented within your assignment is just as important. This will inform the reader whether you have understood the information and where you have looked for it. Referencing Wikipedia is therefore not good practice as it means that you have not looked very far or read any of the original work. If you do use Wikipedia as a starting point you must also read and reference the original article or book.

For some assignments you may be expected to have carried out a literature review (see *Chapter 3*). This usually means a search of available information on evidence-based practice and research. Ellis (2013) suggests that evidence-based practice can mean anything from research to individual stories, so it is important to be able to understand what it is you are reviewing. In particular, he suggests that it is always worthwhile searching the 'grey literature', which means projects and studies that have not been published in books or journals but may be found in project reports and dissertations.

6.5 Organising and composing your work

The next stage is to find and record information on the ideas you have identified in your plan. This is not something that is always taught in higher education and has been identified as a barrier for people who enter higher education after the age of 18, who are the first in the family to go to higher education or who are from different cultural backgrounds. The information may be found from journals, books, the internet and/or the media, and this has been discussed in more detail in *Chapters 3* and *4*. However, you will also need to organise your detailed notes somewhere that you can access them easily. This may be in a simple notebook or an electronic source such as RefWorks or EndNote. Again, you will need to become familiar fairly quickly with these programs so that they will be of use to you throughout the course. You may prefer to use an index box system with individual cards for references and notes from sources you have accessed. You will then begin to join all the information together just as you did in the mind map but, this time, it will be joined by paragraphs. It is important that your work makes sense to the reader, as this will inevitably make it easier to read and mark. For research reports you may want to follow a model of information gathering such as the PICO or SPICE (Ellis, 2013) models which are outlined below.

6.5.1 The PICO model

- **P**atient/problem
- **I**ntervention
- **C**omparison
- **O**utcome

6.5.2 The SPICE model

- **S**etting
- **P**erspective
- **I**ntervention
- **C**omparison
- **E**valuation

Whatever method of organisation and composition you choose, you will need to have your work finished in plenty of time for proofreading. This entails checking that your writing is grammatically correct and that there are no spelling errors in the work. You will have realised by now that managing your time is a very good way of staying organised and keeping to your plan – effective time management is discussed in *Chapter 2*.

Some common signs of poor time management include:

- Untidy presentation
- Late submissions
- Frequent extension requests
- Last-minute writing/tutorial requests
- Poor referencing
- Poor grammar
- Lack of proofreading (evident from frequent spelling mistakes).

You may be able to add more to this list, but if you can you probably need to be looking at your own time management skills. There may be problems appearing that you identified at the planning stage but did nothing about, or there may have been unforeseen events over which you had no control. Whatever is interfering with your time management, you need to deal with it sooner rather than later. Falling behind with coursework will put extra pressure and strain upon your already precious time; dealing with problems promptly prevents small problems from getting out of control. Poor time management can also contribute to a poor mark, which is disappointing to everyone, especially if you have worked so hard on the other aspects of writing your assignment. You may have spent too much time on aspects such as finding the evidence or planning, leaving you little time to write the assignment. If this is the case you will need to look again at your deadline checklist in your diary.

When composing your work you will need to look at what level of composition is expected from you. These should relate to the learning outcomes for each assignment. Academic levels are set by the Quality Assurance Agency and are different for each level of study (see *Table 6.2*).

As can be seen from *Table 6.2*, the composition of your work needs to attain at least the level of your study and be able to demonstrate your ability to achieve that level. The levels are deliberately non-specific, but each course tutor should be able to incorporate the level descriptors into the learning outcomes. This is why it is important to check your own work to see if you have achieved them.

Table 6.2 *Levels of higher education study (adapted from the QAA Framework, 2014)*

- Diploma – student demonstrates knowledge and understanding (discussion) of different concepts

- Degree – student demonstrates awareness and critical analysis of evidence-based practice (research)

- Masters – student is able to critically evaluate (synthesise) research methodologies and apply to practice

ACTIVITY 6.3: ORGANISING AND COMPOSING YOUR WORK

If you are not sure how your work should be laid out, go back to a book or journal article that you have used for your assignment. You can develop your own critical analysis skills by asking the following questions.

- How have the author(s) organised their work?
- How have they referenced the information within the text?
- Do they present an argument within the text or is it just describing something?
- Is it the authors' own opinion or have they used research to support their claims?

6.6 Engineering your work and writing reports

You may also need to write your assignment in different formats depending upon what the assignment or examination brief requires, or if you are writing a literature review or a research report. It is therefore important to be aware of the different requirements. However, developing your own writing style is also important and once you have found what you are comfortable with you will be able to develop your own style more successfully throughout your course. Some students are sculptors who shape and change their work carefully as they go along, while others are engineers who build it up into a solid construction with little change (Cottrell, 2013). Your module tutor may also prefer a particular writing style so it would be wise to check with them to see, for example, if you are required to use headings or not, or if they have any other style preferences.

6.6.1 Essay writing

A written assignment should always include an introduction, to tell the reader where you are going with your analysis, and a conclusion to tell the reader where you have been. The introduction and conclusion are not the same, however, and each should justify their own existence by saying why you have chosen to focus upon a particular area, and conclude with what you have learned during the process. This demonstrates that you have understood the brief and have done your best to answer it within the parameters of the word/time length of the assignment/exam. Most essay-style assignments require the following to be clearly demonstrated:

- Introduction – say what you are going to write about including the module learning outcomes
- Main body – discuss your topic area in as much depth (analysis) as possible
- Conclusion – demonstrate how your knowledge has developed – do not summarise the essay.

6.6.2 Report writing

Writing a report is slightly different from an assignment or exam in that, depending upon the type of report, you will be required to include certain headings. With a research report, for example, you are expected to include the following information.

- Title
- Abstract

- Introduction and background information
- Literature review
- Methods of data collection and analysis
- Results
- Discussion
- Limitations
- Conclusion
- Acknowledgements.

This is a fairly standardised approach to writing reports that many tutors and examiners would expect to see within the assignment (Ellis, 2013). However, it is only likely that you will be required to complete this type of report when you are studying at degree level and above. In all types of writing, your marks will reflect the *presentation, referencing, organisation, composition, engineering, spelling and structure* of the assignment, whatever level you are studying at.

HELPFUL HINT

Remember the PROCESS framework and use this to check your work before you submit it. You can also practise using it on the work of other authors to help you become more aware of the quality and effectiveness of the literature you are reading, e.g. consider the PROCESS framework in the following examples:
- Self-help websites
- Policy and law documents
- National and international guidelines
- Newspaper reports
- Blogs and e-books
- Books and journals.

ACTIVITY 6.4: OBTAINING FEEDBACK

Obtaining feedback and feed-forward (Cottrell, 2013) is a very important part of the learning process but, unfortunately, it is not used to the best advantage. Spend a few minutes thinking about when you last obtained feedback on something that you did well or not so well and how it made you feel about your learning. Also think about any formative assessments you have undertaken (a tutorial can be included in this). Were you given feedback on how to improve your mark and, more importantly, did you use it?

6.7 Spelling and structure

The course tutors usually provide marking guidelines so that students can see what their work will be marked against – this is different from the assignment brief. Some are very elaborate, with each section broken down into individual marks, while others are what are known as grade related, where the marker is free to mark within the grade. If you are provided with marking guidelines, please use them to assess your own standard of work. Some students are now being asked to assess some part of their work themselves and, by becoming their own critic, they can learn how to develop some of their weaker academic writing skills. However, marking guidelines are simply that – guidelines – and they cannot really demonstrate the complex decision-making that takes place when lecturers assess your work. Spelling and structure, however, can contribute to any early impressions a marker will make when reading your work as they will quickly inform the reader that the student may have poor time management skills and poor self-analysis skills.

HELPFUL HINT

When planning your work always allow time for proofreading so that you can find spelling and grammar mistakes before you submit your work. You would think with modern technology this would not be so much of a problem, but it is probably more of a problem now, as many computers and tablets will offer a *predictive text* service and change the word to what it predicts it should be. This can cause a great deal of embarrassment if not checked. To help you proofread your work, try the following tips before you next submit your assignment and you could improve your marks greatly using these simple techniques:

- Avoid long sentences as these can be difficult to read and make sense of
- Use one paragraph for each idea so you can analyse it in more depth
- Read your work to yourself out loud
- Ask a friend or family member to read your work
- Think of the reader/marker as someone who knows nothing about the topic so that you will explain everything clearly
- Never assume that the reader knows what you mean
- Explain every new term the first time you use it, e.g. Health and/or Social Care
- When using definitions use professional evidence-based sources, not dictionaries
- Avoid too many quotations as these can take up valuable word space and always need explaining.

6.7.1 Using marking guidelines to check your spelling and structure

Along with many module tutors, Boore and Deeny (2012) suggest that students can use the marking guidelines to check the level of their spelling and structure. You will find marking guidelines in all of your module handbooks and the marker will also be using these to guide their marking. If a marking rubric is used by the marking tutor it will always be related to the module marking guidelines. The examples below demonstrate how marking guidelines might look in your course, but each university or college will have a slightly different structure.

A-Grade work would include very good grammar and no spelling mistakes, e.g. all paragraphs would discuss ideas presented by the student in depth and flow well throughout the assignment.

B-Grade work would include good grammar with one or two spelling mistakes, e.g. work has been presented in paragraphs (structure) but some spelling mistakes interrupt the flow of the work.

C-Grade work would include some poor grammar and some spelling mistakes, e.g. some sentences are not included in paragraphs (structure) and are too long, making it difficult to read and mark.

D-Grade work would be difficult to read because of poor grammar and spelling, e.g. too many lists or direct quotations used (structure) that do not demonstrate student understanding well.

E/F/Failed work would include very poor grammar, a lot of spelling mistakes and many errors in the structure, e.g. poor sentence construction and spelling, demonstrating lack of proofreading and rushed work.

It is argued that lecturers should be more flexible in setting assessments to accommodate the different needs of students, but in reality, and mainly due to time constraints, the written word is still the main area of assessment. However, this should not be seen as a simple measurement of achievement, i.e. if I do this and that I will get an A, but a complex judgement of the whole piece of work that accumulates throughout the programme of study (Cottrell, 2013). Tutorials with your tutor are therefore very important if you want to achieve the best possible grade or mark, as they will be able to give you their professional advice and opinion on your work. This may include advice on explaining a term in more depth or making sure you have supported your work from the literature you have read. It is very easy to become so immersed in your work that you miss the point of demonstrating your understanding rather than expecting the reader to guess whether you truly understand a concept.

6.7.2 Writing in the first or third person

Students are often confused about whether they should write in the first or third person. When writing in the first person the work in general is usually accepted as being less formal. In this book we have written in the first person to generate a feeling of informality with you, the student. This style of writing is often used in books or where a more personal relationship needs to be developed to get your message across. It does not depend upon the level of study; many doctoral students use the first person when talking about their research.

However, if the work is a more formal piece, then writing in the third person is more appropriate. This means that we do not write about me or you (first or second person) but about people, subjects, participants, authors (the third person) who are less familiar to us. It also demonstrates an ability to be objective within our writing, instead of subjective, and helps us move away from our own opinions towards theoretically informed discussion and analysis. There are therefore arguments for using either first- or third-person writing, but a general rule is that if you are writing about your own experience use 'I' but if not, use 'the author'.

6.8 **Conclusion**

Students who are embarking upon a period of study need to learn the process very quickly and this can be daunting, even for those whose family and/or friends have already been through the process. This chapter has outlined the assessment process of assignments, report writing and examinations in relation to the levels of study within a programme. However, you will need to develop individual skills in planning, gathering and organising information, and managing your own time alongside this process. With some careful preparation and support from the people in place to help, you should quickly become familiar with this new language and feel comfortable in discussing your own needs with tutors and peers.

SUMMARY

Five key points to take away from *Chapter 6*:
- ☑ A plan is the best way to begin your writing and guide your study time.
- ☑ Using your referenced material wisely demonstrates good understanding.
- ☑ Organising and composing your work correctly will help you meet that deadline.
- ☑ Engineering your writing style will develop your academic writing skills.
- ☑ The spelling and structure of your work gives an overall impression of your ability.

Quiz

1. Which one of the following does the PROCESS framework stand for?
   a. Preparation, Referencing, Organisation, Culture, Engineering, Spelling and Structure
   b. Planning, Referencing, Organisation, Composition, Education, Spelling and Structure
   c. Preparation, Research, Organisation, Culture, Education, Spelling and Structure
   d. Planning, Referencing, Organisation, Composition, Engineering, Spelling and Structure

2. Why is it important to proof-read your work? Choose one of the following options
   a. To check the word limit allocated to the assignment
   b. To check the referencing within the assignment
   c. To check the spelling and structure within the assignment
   d. To check the module learning outcomes for the assignment

3. Which one of the following does PICO stand for?
   a. Perspective, Intervention, Comparison, Outcome
   b. Person, Intervention, Composition, Outcome
   c. Perspective, Interpretation, Comparison, Outcome
   d. Perspective, Intervention, Control, Outcome

4. What are marking guidelines used for? Choose one of the following options
   a. To help the marker grade your assignment
   b. To help you grade your assignment
   c. To assess the module learning outcomes within your work
   d. All of the above

REFERENCES

Boore, J. and Deeny, P. (2012) *Nursing Education: planning and delivering the curriculum*. SAGE.

Cottrell, S. (2013) *The Study Skills Handbook*. Macmillan International Higher Education.

Ellis, P. (2013) *Understanding Research for Nursing Students*. Learning Matters.

Lloyd, M. (2007) Developing academic writing skills: the process framework. *Nursing Standard*, 21(40), 50–56.

QAA (2014) *Framework for Higher Education*. Quality Assurance Agency.

Chapter 7
Referencing skills

Helen Thomas, Jacqui Maung, Ella Turner and Paul Verlander

LEARNING OUTCOMES

When you have completed this chapter you should be able to:

7.1 Understand the importance of referencing in relation to academic integrity

7.2 Understand the key principles of producing accurate references regardless of which referencing system you are required to use

7.3 Use different techniques to effectively document and acknowledge your sources.

7.1 Referencing and academic integrity

As a Health and Social Care student, you are not only a part of a community of health practitioners, you are also part of an academic community. Both communities will share some core ethical values, such as respect, honesty, trust and rigour. These are the values of integrity that underpin your academic and professional culture. In your professional life, for example, you would respect another person's physical possessions; you would be honest in your professional opinions, which may be based on rigorous investigation and consultation with patients and fellow colleagues; and you would build trust through that professionalism by acknowledging to others how you have reached your professional judgement.

This is no different from the way you should operate in your academic community: you would respect another person's intellectual property by not stealing their ideas; you would be honest in your academic opinions, which would be based on rigorous investigation of a wide range of academic sources; and you would build trust by acknowledging to your reader how you have reached your judgement and conclusions, by citing the work of others.

You will no doubt already be aware of the importance of evidence-based healthcare as fundamental to your future professional practice. Referencing, the process of acknowledging the sources you have used, is your means of demonstrating that your academic work is based on sound evidence.

IMPROVING RESILIENCE, LIFELONG LEARNING AND EMPLOYABILITY

In your professional practice, although you may not be required to produce academic references, you will, however, have to continually acknowledge the sources of evidence that have informed your decisions and provide an audit trail as to how you have reached clinical decisions. The principles of referencing, acknowledging the sources you have used, is a skill that you will use throughout your working life.

ACTIVITY 7.1

You submit an assignment in your final year of study that is awarded an outstanding first-class grade of 85%. You are very proud as you have worked extremely hard for it.

A year after graduation, you are studying part-time for an MA and you come across a newly published journal article that contains passages that are, word for word, identical to those of your own work from your undergraduate assignment. This article has been written by your former lecturer and contains no acknowledgement or reference to your work.

Discussion points:
1. How would this make you feel?
2. What could the lecturer who wrote the article have done differently?
3. What form of academic malpractice do you think is represented in this scenario?

If you were the student in this scenario, you may feel cheated, hurt or angry. Hopefully, you would feel quite differently if your lecturer had acknowledged your hard work in their article and made some effort to interpret your work in their own words. By citing and paraphrasing your work correctly, the lecturer would be giving you due credit for all of your hard work and would have avoided committing plagiarism, which is one form of academic malpractice.

7.2 Plagiarism

Plagiarism can take different forms, from copying someone else's work and passing it off as your own to colluding with another student to produce and submit the same work (collusion). However, there are other, perhaps more subtle forms of plagiarism that are usually unintentional, such as failing to distinguish between direct quotes and paraphrases, or patchworking (also known as mosaic plagiarism), where your writing will contain fragments of your own 'voice' or language and other unacknowledged phrases from one or more sources. This form of plagiarism is more common and is usually unintentional, often stemming from a lack of understanding about why we need to reference, or from bad writing habits, such as poor planning, note-taking and research.

Whether it is intentional or unintentional makes little difference to the outcome – you will still be held accountable through your institution's policy on plagiarism, where the consequences can vary, depending on the context of the breach of academic integrity.

So, being able to maintain academic integrity and avoid the pitfalls of plagiarism is about much more than the simple mechanics of referencing. Rather than worrying about where to put the commas and the full stops in your list of references, you first need to appreciate how knowledge is constructed in your discipline and develop the skills and confidence in your academic reading and writing.

ACTIVITY 7.2

Below are a set of statements from students containing reasons given for plagiarism. Read each statement carefully and think about the possible explanations behind each reason. How would you advise a student in each situation?

1. 'I panicked – I've been so busy and it was all last minute.'
2. 'I tend to have a webpage open and then copy and paste the bits I need into my Word document, then change some of the words.'
3. 'This was a group project, so my friend and I worked together to complete the assignment.'
4. 'I got mixed up with my notes and couldn't find where I got the information from.'

To develop good academic practice and maintain academic integrity, you need to improve the following skills:

- Time and task management
- Reading and note-taking
- Paraphrasing, summarising, quoting and citations
- Referencing.

You should develop these fundamental skills during your first year at university. This chapter will now go on to examine each skill area in more detail and discuss how their development will help you to maintain academic integrity.

7.3 Developing a rigorous approach to referencing

As we will see, developing effective referencing skills requires planning, organisation and a rigorous approach. In order to reference effectively, you need to think about the requirements of referencing your sources at the very start of preparations for your written work. Good referencing cannot be achieved as an afterthought. Good referencing is based on a rigorous approach to time and task management, to reading and note-taking and to documenting your sources.

7.3.1 Time and task management

Leaving your assignment until the day before the deadline is full of risk, as there are a number of steps involved in the assignment writing process before you should commit anything to paper. Many students fall into the plagiarism trap due to poor planning. Effective planning will give you space to think about what you are going to say, how you are going to say it and what you need to do to be able to say it. Remember that constructing your assignment is like constructing a house – you wouldn't start by laying the bricks. You would need to plan the layout, have a target completion date, choose the right materials and lay foundations. This all takes time!

In order to give yourself time, don't wait until the last lecture on your topic – *you can start as soon as you are given your assignment brief.* Start by reading and deconstructing the assignment title to identify how you are going to approach the answer, the keywords that tell you what the topic is about and any limiting factors, such as the deadline and word count. This will help you to establish what you think you know about the topic and what gaps there are in your knowledge. From this you can complete a diary to set deadlines, starting with the assignment deadline and working backwards. You may prefer to use a large wall-planner, a paper or an online diary, colour-coded so you can clearly prioritise each of your activities. I use an online calendar in my working life to keep track of tasks, so these strategies are important for both your academic and professional roles. See *Chapter 2* for more information about effective time management.

Following the deconstruction of your brief, you can use the key topic words you identified to do a brainstorm, identifying alternative terms (synonyms) that can inform your library search strategy. Once you have completed preliminary reading, you can revisit your brainstorm and begin to draft another to plan the structure of your assignment, based on your initial reading.

7.3.2 Reading and note-taking

Your knowledge is built from the knowledge of others and from your experiences. In your degree you are expected to read the ideas of others to add to and extend your knowledge, as well as practically apply that knowledge to shape and build your experience, which can further inform your reflections on your practice.

Therefore, you should aim to read a variety of academic sources, including books and journal articles, to obtain a range of scholarly opinions on your topic from which you can form your own judgements. The more recently published sources will contain the most up-to-date evidence in your field. Think critically about the extent to which currency of information impacts on how relevant it is to your topic. In all health and social care disciplines research, treatments, therapies, policy and legislation change over time. Thinking about currency of information can help you filter out irrelevant material when you conduct your search.

You will find more information about reading and note-taking in *Chapter 3*, but in relation to referencing it is particularly important to make a note of your sources. When you find a relevant source, at the time you first use it, note down everything you need to find the source again – this will form your reference for your assignment. Documenting the information you will need to reference sources as part of the note-taking process will save a considerable amount of time and effort when you come to prepare your references. Or to put things another way, if you don't document the information you will need to reference your sources when note-taking, you will find yourself in a scenario like this:

SCENARIO 7.1

You think you have completed a 5000-word essay and are now doing your references after a final proofread. You realise that you need to add in citations to quotes you have used. Because you didn't do so when originally making notes, you now need to revisit all the books you have used, note down all the details of those books for your reference list and find out where in the books your quotations appeared. Furthermore, you have already had to return some of those books to the library and you now find some of them are out on loan to other students. In addition, you have used some journal articles but you cannot remember where you downloaded them from. You also used a government document from the web but when you Google it again, you cannot find it.

The above scenario will undoubtedly lead to several more hours of work and likely lost marks for incomplete references which with a bit of planning could easily have been avoided.

 IMPROVING RESILIENCE, LIFELONG LEARNING AND EMPLOYABILITY

Developing a rigorous approach to referencing will build your resilience and help you to avoid situations such as that in *Scenario 7.1*.

Irrespective of which referencing system your university requires you to use, the elements you will need to note down for most sources will be the same. The following section provides more details on how to locate this information in different kinds of sources.

Note down the information you will need to reference the source at the top of your page/index card or referencing app, or whatever system you are using to manage your information. Underneath this, you can then make your notes in your own words and include a page number (if using a source that includes page numbers) so you can find exactly where you found this information. You may also find it helpful to highlight direct quotes in a different colour, as a clear reminder in your notes that you need to distinguish between your own voice and that of the author's.

7.3.3 Documenting your sources

Books

For books you should document the following information:

- The full title of the book as appears on the title page (including any subtitle)
- The full names of the author(s) or editor(s) as listed on the title page
- The date the book was published
- The publishing company the book was published by
- Where the book was published (in other words, where the publishing company is based)
- The edition of the book.

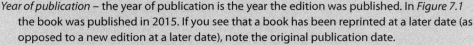

HELPFUL HINTS ✔

Year of publication – the year of publication is the year the edition was published. In *Figure 7.1* the book was published in 2015. If you see that a book has been reprinted at a later date (as opposed to a new edition at a later date), note the original publication date.

Editions – unless a book states an edition number, assume it is the first edition. Just because a book has been reprinted does not mean that it is a new edition.

Place of publication – if the publishing company has offices in several different places note down the first location listed. Include the country as well as the place name.

Edited books – *Figure 7.1* is an extract from an edited book. In other words, the book will have been compiled by one or more editors but each chapter will be written by different authors. As well as the title of the book and the editor details, for each chapter that you have used, note down the author(s) and title of the chapter as well. Also note down the start page and end page of each chapter you have used.

E-books – note down name of the e-book provider from which you accessed the book and the website address where the book was found. Also note down the date that you accessed the e-book. Some referencing systems may require this information.

Journal articles

For journal articles you should document the following information:

- The author(s) of the article
- The title of the article
- The name of the journal the article was published in
- The year the issue of the journal was published
- The volume number and issue number of the journal issue the article appeared in
- The page numbers within the issue that the article appeared in

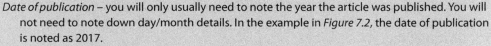

HELPFUL HINTS ✔

Date of publication – you will only usually need to note the year the article was published. You will not need to note down day/month details. In the example in *Figure 7.2*, the date of publication is noted as 2017.

Issue details – sometimes it may not be clear which is the volume number and which is the issue number. If two numbers are quoted following the name of the journal, the first will be the volume number and the second the issue number. In the example shown in *Figure 7.2* the issue details are volume 54, number 4.

Identifying page numbers – if these are not listed at the top of the article, use the pagination at the bottom of the pages.

Author names – be sure to note down the names of all authors of the article. You do not need to note down details of which organisations the authors are from.

Online journal articles – note down the DOI (which stands for digital object identifier) of the article if you can see one identified. If you can't see a DOI note down the web address where you found the article. Also note down the date that you accessed the journal article. Some referencing systems may require this information.

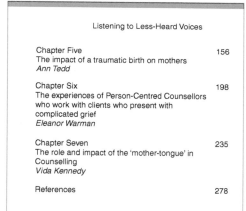

Listening to Less-Heard Voices:

Developing Counsellors' Awareness

Edited by

Peter Madsen Gubi

University of Chester Press

First published 2015
by University of Chester Press
University of Chester
Parkgate Road
Chester CH1 4BJ

Printed and bound in the UK by the
LIS Print Unit
University of Chester
Cover designed by the
LIS Graphics Team
University of Chester

The introduction and editorial material
© University of Chester, 2015
The individual chapters
© the respective authors, 2015

A catalogue record for this book is available from the British
Library

ISBN 978-1-908258-23-6

Listening to Less-Heard Voices

Figure 7.1 *Preliminary pages of a sample book provide information needed for referencing.*
Copyright University of Chester Press. Reproduced with permission.

International Journal of Study Skills Vol. 54(4), August 2017, 547–582
© Study Skills Publishing

Students' Referencing Skills as They Impact on Anxiety Levels and Overall Well-being: a Case Study of Health and Social Care Students at a UK University

Sarah G. Smith
University of Chester
Gordon P. Jones
Bangor University

Abstract

Lack of ability in referencing and the negative impact this may have on academic attainment has long been thought to be a contributory factor to student stress and anxiety levels at times close to assessment submission. However, to date evidence has largely been anecdotal and based on reflections of individual students.

Introduction

_____
_____
_____
_____
_____
_____
_____
_____
_____
_____
_____

Figure 7.2 *The information needed to cite a journal.*

Online sources of information

In addition to e-books and online journal articles, there is a very wide range of other material that you find on the free web (or from subscription sites) that you may find yourself using when researching your written work. This includes things such as:

- Web pages from relevant websites (for example, information on NHS and Department of Health sites)
- Reports and documents that you have downloaded from the free web (for example, NHS policy documents, research written by government bodies)
- Legislation that you have accessed online.

Whenever you use sources that you access online, it is good practice to always note down the following information. Depending on the referencing system you are using, you may need this information to acknowledge the fact that it is an online version you are using when you come to produce your reference list:

- The full title of the web page or document
- The full address of the site where the information was found
- Any names of individual authors that are listed on the page or document
- The name of the organisation
- The date you visited the site where you found the page/document.

HELPFUL HINTS

Use your judgement – referencing online sources often requires exercising judgement/interpretation, but as a rule of thumb note down all the information available that will help you attribute the source and someone else to find it.

Web addresses – note down the exact web address of the page (or where the document can be downloaded) as highlighted in *Figures 7.3* and *7.4*.

Title – In the case of PDF documents such as in *Figure 7.3* the title may be relatively clear. However, in the case of a web page such as *Figure 7.4* it may be less so. In the case of web pages, include whatever is the main header of the page as your title.

Author(s) – if no individual authors are identified, note down the name of the organisation that produced the information.

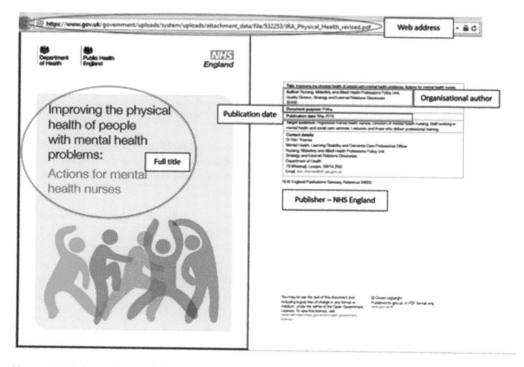

Figure 7.3 *Information needed to cite a pdf source.*
© Crown Copyright 2016

Publisher – information on web pages may be more limited. In the case of *Figure 7.3* both an organisational author and a publisher are identified. In *Figure 7.4* the only author/publisher information is NHS.

Publication date – in the case of PDF documents such as *Figure 7.3* a clear publication date may be identified. In *Figure 7.4* this isn't the case. Remember a 'page updated' or 'page reviewed' date is not the same as a publication date. If you can't see a publication date, note down that the source does not have a date. Most referencing systems will have particular rules for documenting undated sources.

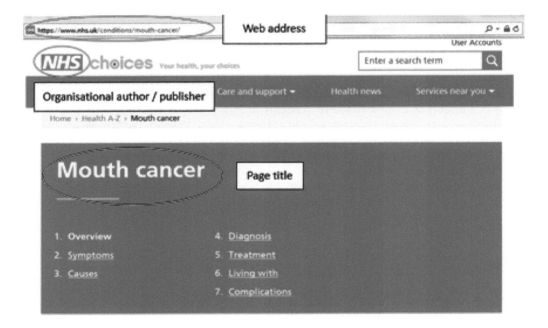

Figure 7.4 *Information needed to cite an internet resource.*
© C rown Copyright 2016

ACTIVITY 7.3

Remember, an important part of avoiding plagiarism is being organised. So take this opportunity to decide how you are going to organise your notes from your reading. Try organising your notes alphabetically, using the authors' surnames. If you are using card indexes to write your notes on, invest in a card index holder to organise them. If you are using paper, or a Word document on your PC, then create a literature folder and subfolders, renaming each subfolder to a letter of the alphabet to organise your notes alphabetically. Alternatively, you may find it easier to organise your notes by themes in your assignment, which is fine, as long as you use a method that works for you.

7.4 **Referencing**

Once you understand the principles of why it is important to acknowledge your sources and how to document your sources as you research your written work, you are now in a position to use your sources within your written work. As we will see shortly, while there are many different styles of referencing in different referencing systems, the fundamental principles of how to paraphrase, summarise, quote, cite and the mechanics of producing references will be the same throughout your academic career.

7.4.1 Paraphrasing, summarising, quoting and citations

When you make your notes, they should be in your own words. Even if you think they don't read as well, using your own words will count for more. Committing plagiarism is serious, so it's better to lose a few marks for poor academic style, as this is something that can be developed, whereas an accusation of plagiarism could result in failure of the assignment or worse.

Being able to paraphrase, summarise and quote correctly are essential skills for becoming a successful assignment writer.

What makes a good summary?

- Condense lengthy information and present in a concise form
- Focus on giving the key ideas or main points
- Retain the original meaning.

To get started on summarising:
- Read the text several times until you clearly understand the meaning
- Highlight the key points
- Make a note in bullet form of the key points in your own words
- Now write the summary directly from these notes, without looking at the original text
- Check the summary against the original to ensure that it is an accurate reflection of the author's ideas.

What makes a good paraphrase?

- Attempt to restate the relevant ideas of an author using your own words
- Change the wording *and* the structure
- Retain the original meaning.

To get started on paraphrasing:
- Read the text several times until you clearly understand the meaning
- Underline any words that can be changed
- Find other words or phrases that have similar meanings to those you have underlined (synonyms)
- Change the word order
- Check your paraphrase against the original to ensure that it is an accurate reflection of the author's ideas.

How do I quote effectively?

- Use the original words of the author
- Do not over-use quotations
- Think about the point you want to make with the quote
- Keep the quote as concise as possible.

What is a citation?

Whether you are paraphrasing, summarising or directly quoting from a source, in the body of your written work you will need to include details of the source this information has come from. We call this the citation, and including a citation is part of the process of referencing. The following section will now explain the principles of producing citations and references.

7.4.2 Different referencing systems

All written work at university level will require you to use a referencing system to acknowledge sources you have used. Unfortunately, there is no universal method of referencing; rather, there are several different systems, many of which may also be subject to variation between different universities, or even departments and faculties within universities. The referencing system you are required to use will therefore depend on where you are studying.

Some referencing systems, such as Harvard and the American Psychological Association (APA) referencing system, are based upon using an author/date citation within the body of your text whenever you refer to a source you have used. Other systems such as MHRA (commonly used in humanities subjects) make use of footnotes at the bottom of each page which note full references to sources. The Vancouver referencing system (often used in the physical sciences), instead of citing the author and date of a source within your text, will indicate a source has been used by placing a number. These numbers will then correspond to numbered references in a referencing list.

It is important that before you start you check which referencing system your department uses and make sure you follow the guidance produced on that referencing system.

How to reference

Examples follow which illustrate the principles of doing your references in academic work. The examples shown use the American Psychological Association (APA) referencing system. However, regardless of which referencing system you are using, the elements of information you will need to reference different kinds of sources will be the same.

When referencing your sources you will need to produce your reference in two ways:
1. In-text citation: as discussed in the previous section, citation is the process of acknow-ledging the work you have directly referred to in the body of your text. In the APA system this will involve noting the surname of the author(s) and date of the publication you are referencing.
2. In the Reference list: create a list of references at the end of your text with full details of the works you have referred to in your text.

Each of your citations within the body of your text must correspond accurately to the one in the list of references at the end.

Bibliographies

In addition to a reference list, some referencing systems may also require you to produce a bibliography. This is a list of everything that you read in order to produce your written assignment, irrespective of whether or not you directly referred to that source in your writing. Below is a range of different sources that are commonly used in assignments. Each source type is recreated in an APA referencing style – other systems will require similar information but in a slightly different format.

Printed books

Figure 7.5 shows an image from the first few pages of a printed book which has two authors. The elements that you need to use to create a reference were mentioned earlier in this chapter. To create a printed book reference you will need to include the full title of the book, including any subtitles, the full name(s) of the author(s), the date the book was published, the publisher and the place of publication. All this information can be found on the front pages of a printed book.

**Advocacy and
Public Speaking:**

A Student's Introduction

Derek Halbert and Hayley Whitaker
University of Chester Law School, 2016

With a Foreword by
**The Rt Hon. the Lord Thomas
of Cwmgiedd Kt, PC**
Lord Chief Justice of England and Wales

University of Chester Press

First published 2016
by University of Chester Press
Parkgate Road
Chester CH1 4BJ

Printed and bound in the UK by the
LIS Print Unit
University of Chester
Cover designed by the LIS Graphics Team
University of Chester

© Hayley Whitaker and Derek Halbert, 2016
Foreword © The Rt Hon. the Lord Thomas
of Cwmgiedd Kt, PC, 2016

All Rights Reserved
No part of this publication may be reproduced, stored
in a retrieval system or transmitted in any form or
by any means without the prior permission of the
copyright owner, other than as permitted by UK
copyright legislation or under the terms and
conditions of a recognised copyright licensing scheme

A catalogue record of this book is available
from the British Library

ISBN 978-1-908258-27-4

Figure 7.5 *Example of the preliminary pages of a multi-author publication.*
Copyright University of Chester Press. Reproduced with permission.

The following is how this would look in an APA reference list:
Halbert, D., & Whitaker, H. (2016). Advocacy and public speaking: A student's introduction. Chester, United Kingdom: University of Chester Press.

In-text citation

When you want to acknowledge the book in the main body of your assignment, you will need to create an in-text citation which flags to the reader that you are referring to someone else's work. The precise style of in-text citation will depend upon the referencing system you are using; for example, using APA the above book would be cited as:
Halbert and Whitaker (2016) argued that …

For more information about in-text citations, see the citation tips section at the end of the chapter.

Looking back at *Figure 7.1*, you will see it is an example of an edited book with chapters written by different authors. If you want to reference a particular chapter, commonly used referencing systems will expect you to record the author, title and page numbers of the chapter within the book that you have used as well as the details of the book itself.

The following is an example of how a chapter from the book shown in *Figure 7.1* would look in an APA reference list:

Todd, A. (2015). The impact of a traumatic birth on mothers. In P. M. Gubi (Ed.), Listening to Less-Heard Voices: Developing counsellors' awareness (pp. 156–197). Chester, United Kingdom: University of Chester Press.

The in-text citation in APA style would look like this:
According to Todd (2015) …

Different editions of books

It is always important to use the most up-to-date edition of any book as often authors' opinions may be revised, or in the case of clinical procedures information may be updated to reflect current knowledge and professional regulations. As we have seen earlier, this information is always present in the publication detail pages within the book.

When referencing your work, you should always include the edition in your reference if there has been more than one edition of the book to indicate that you are using the most up-to-date edition and to flag which edition you have read.

The following is an example of how this would look in an APA reference list:
Dimond, B. (2015). Legal Aspects of Nursing. (7th ed.). Harlow, United Kingdom: Pearson.

The in-text citation in APA style would look like this:
According to Dimond (2015) …

E-books

If you have used an e-book in your work you must distinguish between this format and a print version. The information required for an e-book reference is similar to that for a printed book, but instead of publication information you need to note the website address of the e-book provider from which you accessed the book. You should also note down the date you accessed the e-book, as some referencing systems may require this.

The printed book with authors we used as an example in *Figure 7.5* is also available in online format, provided by e-book provider Dawson Era.

The following is an example of how this would look in an APA reference list:
Halbert, D., & Whitaker, H. (2016). Advocacy and Public Speaking: A student's introduction. Retrieved from https://www.dawsonera.com

The in-text citation in APA style would look like this:
Research by Halbert and Whitaker (2016) showed …

Journal articles, print and online

As a student of Health and Social Care you will need to ensure that the information you are using for your studies is up to date. One of the best ways of finding recent research is by using journal articles. Most journals are available in both print and online formats, and just as with books, it is important to distinguish between the two formats in your references.

Printed journal article

When you have used a printed article is it important to make a note of the following: the author(s) and full title of the article, the name of the journal the article was published in, the year the issue was published, volume and issue number and the article page numbers.

The following is an example of how this would look in an APA reference list:
Brown, A., Rance, J., & Bennett, P. (2015). Understanding the relationship between breast-feeding and postnatal depression: The role of pain and physical difficulties. Journal of Advanced Nursing, 72(2), 273–282.

The in-text citation in APA style would look like this:
This conclusion is supported by research reported in Brown, Rance and Bennett (2015).

Online journal article

You also need to distinguish between print and online versions of an article when referencing. The information required for an online article reference is similar to that for a printed article, with the addition of a DOI (digital object identifier). You also may be required to note down the date you accessed the article as some referencing systems may require this. If you cannot find a DOI present you will need to note the website address of the journal homepage in your reference.

The following is an example of how this would look in an APA reference list:
Brown, A., Rance, J., & Bennett, P. (2015). Understanding the relationship between breast-feeding and postnatal depression: The role of pain and physical difficulties. Journal of Advanced Nursing, 72(2), 273–282. https://doi.org/10.1111/jan.12832

The in-text citation in APA style would look like this:
This conclusion is supported by research reported in Brown, Rance and Bennett (2015).

Online documents and reports

Always make sure you note down the date you visited the website where you found the document as web pages are liable to change over time. For this reference we will use the example of an online report used in *Figure 7.3*. The information you will need includes the following: full title of the web page or document, full address of the website, names of authors that are listed on the page, the name of the organisation and the date you accessed the document online, as some referencing systems may require this.

The following is an example of how this would look in an APA reference list:

Nursing, Midwifery and Allied Health Professionals Policy Unit, Quality Division, Strategy and External Relations Directorate. (2016). Improving the physical health of people with mental health problems: Actions for mental health nurses. Retrieved from https://www.gov.uk/government/uploads/system/uploads/attachment_data/file/532253/JRA_Physical_Health_revised.pdf

The in-text citation in APA style would look like this:

According to a report published in 2016 … (Nursing, Midwifery and Allied Health Professionals Policy Unit, Quality Division, Strategy and External Relations Directorate).

Online document without a date of publication

Sometimes the date of publication is not shown on a web page, as shown in *Figure 7.4*. In this case you will need to note in your reference that there is no publication date given. The format for recording this in your reference will vary according to the referencing system you are using. You will also need to note the full title of the web page or document, the full web address from where you retrieved the document, any names of authors listed, the name of the organisation and the date you visited the website.

The following is an example of how this would look in an APA reference list:

NHS Choices. (n.d.). Mouth cancer. Retrieved February 27, 2018 from https://www.nhs.uk/conditions/mouth-cancer/

The in-text citation in APA style would look like this:

Guidance given by NHS Choices (n.d.) advises the following …

HELPFUL HINT

Where information is missing, such as the date the information was produced, think carefully about whether it is still appropriate to refer to this source. For example, if you cannot tell when the information is published it could be out of date, which as we know is particularly problematic for a subject area like health and social care.

Images

Depending on the subject of your assignment you may wish to refer to an image you have consulted, such as a diagram from a book or a website. The information you will need to note down for your reference may include the following: creator of the image, date the image was created, title of the image, the format used (for example photograph) and the web address of the page where you accessed the image. You should also note the date you accessed the image if found online, as you may be required to record this in your reference.

The following is an example of how an image from an online source would look in an APA reference list:

Gathany, J. (2010). *Anopheles gambiae* [Photograph]. Retrieved from http://hardinmd.lib.uiowa.edu/cdc/malaria3.html

The in-text citation in APA style would look like this:
Gathany's photograph (2010) shows a mosquito feeding …

Systematic review

A Cochrane systematic review is a balanced and impartial summary of all the available research evidence, published and unpublished, carried out on a specific health topic. When you read a Cochrane systematic review you need to note down the following elements that you may be required to use to create your reference: the author(s) of the review, year of publication, title of the review, volume and issue number, page numbers, the DOI and the date you accessed the review.

The following is an example of how a Cochrane Systematic Review would look in an APA reference list:
Wiffen, P. J., Wee, B., & Moore, R. A. (2016). Oral morphine for cancer pain. Cochrane Database of Systematic Reviews, 2016(4), 1–104. https:// doi.org/10.1002/14651858.CD003868. pub4

The in-text citation in APA style would look like this:
Oral morphine is widely used to help relieve severe cancer pain (Wiffen, Wee & Moore, 2016).

Secondary citation

You should try wherever possible to locate the original source and cite it directly – by doing this you can ensure that the reference actually supports the point that you are trying to make.

You may find in the course of your reading that you come across a reference to another source which you have not read directly. In this case you would use a secondary citation in your work. A secondary citation is a reference to a source that you have found in another text but which you have not directly consulted yourself. Your reference should be for the work you have actually read, but you will also need to acknowledge in the body of your text the author of the secondary source.

The information you will need to note to create a secondary citation may include the following: name of author(s) whose work you want to reference but have not been able to read, author(s) and title of the source you have read, date of publication of the source, publisher and place of publication if a printed source or web page address/DOI and date when you accessed the source online.

The following example shows a secondary citation to a source by Porter which has been found in a book by Scriven.
Scriven, A. (2017). Ewles & Simnett's Promoting Health: A practical guide. (7th ed.). Edinburgh, United Kingdom: Elsevier.

The following is an example of how this secondary citation would look in an APA reference list:
According to research undertaken by Porter (as cited in Scriven, 2017) …

Use an introductory sentence or phrase before the summary/paraphrase/quote to provide context and add your voice. Try the University of Manchester's Academic Phrasebank for examples: www.phrasebank.manchester.ac.uk

Use both active and passive citations in your writing to improve your academic style:

Active: Verlander (2018) argued that Turner's part of the chapter was the most informative.

Passive: It is widely agreed that Turner's part of the chapter needed significant improvement (Verlander, 2018).

Use reporting verbs to introduce the point you want to make with your summary/paraphrase/quote:

- ☑ Turner (2018) suggests …
- ☑ It is now generally accepted …
- ☑ The latest figures demonstrate …

7.5 **Conclusion**

Referencing your work properly may seem like a hard task, but when done properly and with care it can improve the presentation of your work greatly. When you submit an assignment this is one of the things the marker will look at first and we can tell just from the presentation and reference list where you have looked for information and how you have presented the information. It is worthwhile to start thinking about how you will store information and submit it with your final draft. If you take good care of your reference list it will help you to feel confident about the work you submit and could take your marks into the next grade on the marking criteria.

SUMMARY

Four key points to take away from *Chapter 7*:
- ☑ Good referencing skills improve the quality and presentation of your work.
- ☑ Paraphrasing is an important skill to avoid plagiarism.
- ☑ There are many different ways to reference your sources.
- ☑ Good referencing skills take time to develop.

Quiz

1. Below is a reference for a printed journal. What information is not necessary?
   Ledoux, K. (2015). Understanding compassion fatigue: Understanding compassion. *Journal of Advanced Nursing, 71*(9), 2041–2050. ISSN 03092402.

2. Below is a reference for a printed book. What information is missing?
   Tingle, J., & Cribb, A. (Eds.). (2014). *Nursing Law and Ethics*. (4th ed.).

3. Using your own university's preferred referencing system, try creating a reference using this information for an online article.
   Authors: Darch, J Baillie, L Gillison, F
   Year of publication: 2017
   Article title: Nurses as role models in health promotion: A concept analysis
   Journal title: British Journal of Nursing
   Volume and issue numbers: Vol 27 Issue 17 Pages 982–988
   DOI: https://doi.org/10.12968/bjon.2017.26.

REFERENCE

American Psychological Association (2010) *Publication Manual of the American Psychological Association*, 6th edition. APA.

Chapter 8
Feedback

Peggy Murphy and Craig Morley

LEARNING OUTCOMES

When you have completed this chapter you should be able to:

8.1 Use feedback to take control over your personal and academic development

8.2 Interpret common feedback statements and seek clarification from peers, tutor and others

8.3 Use feedback to create a personal action plan to improve academic performance and percentage grades.

8.1 Introduction

Many students feel disheartened when getting a lower grade than expected, or can become complacent when receiving a high grade. Other students only look at their final grade and do not pay attention to their feedback. Interacting positively with feedback and using feedback effectively is key to improving your marks. Feedback is usually given at the end of a module, following assessment, but with active reflection, feedback can be used as a springboard to help you achieve better grades in future assignments. This chapter will help you regard feedback from others as an opportunity to facilitate your academic growth.

It is inevitable that you will receive positive and negative feedback, both in university and in your career. How you respond to praise and criticism will play a large role in your personal, academic and professional development. To help you think about the importance of feedback and how it can motivate you to improve your studies, this chapter will consider effective approaches to working with feedback for academic development.

8.2 The purpose of feedback

Feedback can take many different forms:
- Formal written feedback following assessments
- Informal verbal feedback from tutors
- Peer-to-peer feedback from fellow students
- Generic group- or cohort-based feedback
- Self-evaluation and reflection.

Feedback is used to highlight what you have done well and what can be improved upon. Constructive feedback enhances student learning. Feedback takes on greater importance when students use it to form a discussion with their marker. To get the most from feedback you need to proactively engage with it. This will enable you to identify goals for your academic and professional development, and help you create action plans to reach those goals.

Hounsell (2004) defines feedback as 'any information, process or activity which affords or accelerates student learning' (p. 1). Feedback is not merely used as a method to rank performance and competency, but as a distinct teaching tool. It is the most common form of guidance university students receive on how to improve their work. As a result, it is important to view feedback as more than a score awarded for a piece of work. Instead, it is more useful to view feedback as a conversation between yourself and your tutor (Nicol and Macfarlane-Dick, 2006; Nicol, 2010). Mortiboys (2005) recognises the emotional dimension within the teacher/learner relationship and that it is beneficial to both to adopt an emotional state that is conducive to learning. Working in partnership with your tutor helps you to gain a sense of control over your own learning rather than being a passive recipient of knowledge.

8.3 Feedback mindset

Your mindset and attitude towards feedback has a direct effect on your ability to utilise it effectively to develop your academic and professional competencies.

Dweck (2006) coined the terms 'fixed mindset' and 'growth mindset'. She recognised that the way you perceive yourself as a learner can have a profound effect on how you develop through life. Dweck (2006) stated that if you believe your abilities are set in stone you are less likely to work through challenges and more likely to see problems as insurmountable. This approach is termed a 'fixed mindset'. People with a 'fixed mindset' believe that intelligence and personality were allotted at birth and that nothing can change that.

Conversely, people with a 'growth mindset' view challenges as learning opportunities and believe in their own ability to develop skills through engaging in problem-solving behaviour. Growth mindset people are prepared to work on their learning. Adopting this approach allows you to perceive feedback from others as a way to help map your progress and develop further. To engage with feedback effectively you should not, therefore, view negative feedback as a failure, but as an opportunity to overcome obstacles and facilitate your own development.

 IMPROVING RESILIENCE, LIFELONG LEARNING AND EMPLOYABILITY

Using feedback effectively to overcome obstacles helps to build motivation and resilience.

Resilience is another quality that students are advised to develop. Resilience, in both an academic and a professional setting, is the ability to recover from difficulties and setbacks. As a student, it is important to develop techniques that motivate you, particularly when you do not get the grades or feedback that you wanted. If you develop the resilience to stick with your programme despite occasional negative feedback you can visualise yourself receiving your certificate at your graduation ceremony. Duckworth (2016) has found that the difference between the best and worst academic performers is not always due to intelligence. She researched what motivates students to learn and found that intelligence quotient (IQ), which only measures whether students learn quickly and easily, is not the best forecast for how students will succeed in life. She found the most important predictor of student success was resilience and grit.

ACTIVITY 8.1: UNDERSTANDING FEEDBACK

Alice has been given feedback on her first assignment at university. She has been awarded 48% for her essay and would like to know how to improve her grades. Look at the following feedback and think about suggestions you could make to her as a peer so you can support her to develop her writing. You could use a SWOT analysis from *Chapter 12* to help her to focus on what she does well and what she needs to improve for her next assignment.

An example of student feedback

Thank you for your work,

It was evident that you have thought about your development in relation to the NMC standards for pre-registration education progression point 2.
Introduction: The signposting of the answer is an important stage in introducing what you will do in the main body of your essay. It was clear that you would include 2 developmental issues that related to progression point 2 of the NMC (2010) standards for education in the main body of your work.
Section 1. It was evident that you had read current literature to inform your action plan as to how you would meet your objectives.
Section 2. The section on building confidence and time management was less organised. It could have been improved with a little more structure and you need to support all of your statements by referring to current literature.
Conclusion: Here again, you would benefit from study skills advice to be able to showcase your thoughts more clearly.
References and supporting literature: Use the APA guide to help you to reference correctly. You would benefit from reading around each topic a little more generally first to get an overview. Also always try to use the author's surname and date of publication in text citations.
Advice for further improvement: This essay demonstrated that you understood the assessment brief. To improve your marks further, try to support all of your statements throughout your work by referring to the literature you have read to inform your ideas. It may benefit you to seek study skills advice on how to structure your work.

8.4 **Feed-forward**

This section will look at the ways in which you can turn feedback into *feed-forward*, as a means to improve grades, as well as maintain motivation and build resilience.

Feed-forward offers students the opportunity to adapt their work using feedback from others before the final submission. The aim of this is that students reflect upon the comments and advice and apply these principles to the whole of their assessment (Butters *et al.*, 2013). In other words, feed-forward is a method used to encourage students to make connections between assessment, feedback and learning. Usually this method involves students presenting a sample of their work to a tutor or study skills advisor for comment. When students are proactive and use this approach they have an opportunity to reflect upon feedback and think about designing their own strategy for success.

Your entire journey as a university student is a formative experience. You are continually asked to learn new skills, knowledge and competencies. To gain the best grades you are capable of, you need to proactively plan your own academic and professional development. Taking responsibility for your own formative learning, by making effective use of feedback from one assignment to the next, is essential in becoming an independent and empowered learner (Boud, 2000). Reflection plays an important role in this. Reflecting on feedback, to identify your strengths and weaknesses, allows you to decide what to do with feedback. Developing reflective practice not only benefits your grades at university, it is a key element of lifelong learning (Fry *et al.*, 2009; Schön, 1987). For that reason, reflecting on your feedback, to decide what study skills and subject knowledge you need to develop, allows you to act as your own source of feed-forward, by using feedback from one assignment to improve your performance in the next.

ACTIVITY 8.2: QUICK REFLECTION

Reflection does not always have to be complex and time-consuming. The simplest reflection is often the most effective reflection. Look back on your last piece of assignment feedback and decide what you are going to:
Stop doing
Start doing
Continue doing.

8.5 Action planning

To get the most from feedback, you will need to formulate a clear response to the advice given. One method is to create an action plan (*Figure 8.1*). Action planning turns passive reflection into active reflection.

Action plans are used to focus reflection and create clearly defined responses to feedback. The setting of goals and the motivation to achieve those goals is a key aspect of becoming an effective independent and lifelong learner (Pintrich and Zusho, 2002). Action planning requires you to create a set of realistic goals to improve the skills that have been identified in your feedback.

The following are examples of different strategies and tactics you may adopt in an action plan:

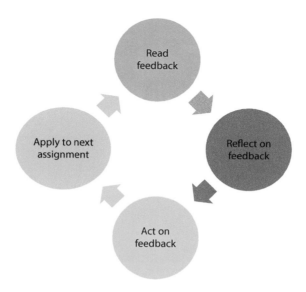

Figure 8.1 *Action plan cycle.*

- Contact study skills team to get help with referencing
- Attend a development seminar (study skills or practical)
- Make an appointment with, or email your tutor to discuss the theory you did not understand
- Create your own glossary of key terms to help define key terminology
- Give yourself more time to proofread assignments in order to spot spelling or grammar mistakes.

Whatever action you take, use SMART targets to formulate your response to feedback. SMART targets are achievable and practical goals (*Figure 8.2*). An open-ended target, such as 'improve my academic writing', is a very broad topic consisting of many different aspects that may be difficult to achieve. To use SMART goals, set specific (S) targets such as 'develop my use of academic language'. Specific targets are easier to measure (M). For example, in your feedback you may notice that you no longer receive comments such as 'too colloquial'. Targets that can be measured and tracked also have the benefit of being more attainable (A) and realistic (R); they are within your power to achieve. It is also important that your goals can be achieved in a timely (T) manner, preferably before your next assignment. In this way, SMART targets help you to make consistent progress that will have a positive effect on future assignments.

 IMPROVING RESILIENCE, LIFELONG LEARNING AND EMPLOYABILITY

When you enter the workforce you will have regular development and performance reviews. Knowing how to use feedback and SMART targets effectively will help you to improve the care you give to the people you are helping and to make good progress in your career.

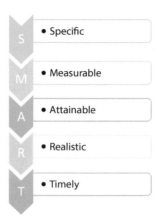

Figure 8.2 *Smart targets.*

ACTIVITY 8.3: SMART TARGETS

Break these broad goals into SMART targets.
'Improve my academic writing'
    1 ....
    2. ....
'Do better in exams'
    1. ....
    2. ....

HELPFUL HINT ✔

After you have created an action plan using SMART, keep it somewhere you can see it every day, perhaps in the bathroom. This will remind you of your targets and help you to stay motivated to achieve them. When you receive your next piece of assignment feedback, check to see if you have achieved your target. If so, cross it off the action plan; that way you can see the progress you are making in your own development.

ACTIVITY 8.4: ACTION PLANNING

1. Look back and reflect on your last piece of assignment feedback.
2. Using the action plan form below, identify which of your study skills are strong and which can be developed further. Mark each skill the feedback mentions from 1 to 5 (1 = weakest, 5 = strongest).
3. Make a plan of how you will develop these skills before your next assignment. (Think about what support services your university has that can help you.)

Take control and ownership of your own development – use feedback to create action plans to aid your own progress.

Action plan form

Time management and organisation	Feedback score
Setting and meeting deadlines	
Prioritising	
Reading and research	
Understanding assignment briefs/essay questions	
Managing reading load	
Using credible and reliable academic sources	
Finding further reading	
Reading texts effectively	
Critical reading/thinking	
Academic writing	
Understanding academic/literary genres	
Quoting, paraphrasing, summarising	
Writing to word count	
Editing – first/second/final drafts	
Academic language	
Critical writing	
Editing/proofreading strategies	
Structure and planning	
Introductions/conclusions	
Creating and sticking to plans	
Paragraph structure	
Organising information	
Making an argument/answering the question	
Academic integrity	
Understanding plagiarism	
Referencing	

Time management and organisation	Feedback score
Action plan **(How will you develop these skills?)**	**By when?**
1.	
2.	
3.	

8.5.1 Feedback glossary

Use this feedback glossary to identify what your tutor says in your feedback, and what they really mean.

What your tutors say	What they mean
'Too colloquial'/ 'Colloquialism'	This means that your writing includes slang, clichés or conversational phrases (e.g. 'the evidence really paints a picture'). Substitute examples of this for more formal language. Academic writing has a specific set of guidelines, styles and conventions. Follow these guidelines closely and consistently in your own writing.
'Reference needed'/ 'Evidence?'	This means that you have not backed up your point with clear evidence, or that you have included a personal judgement that cannot be supported by the evidence. If you are unsure on *how*, *when* or *why* to reference, it is important to seek advice as soon as possible (see *Chapter 7* for more information).
'This is not a credible source'/'More reading of the literature needed'	This means you have not used reliable and credible scholarly and academic reading material. You should always aim to use academic books and journal articles as opposed to newspapers, blogs and online magazines. Conducting effective research is key to gaining high grades in your assignments (see *Chapter 4* for more information).
'Be more critical'/'Go more in-depth'	This means you have not evaluated or analysed the evidence you have used. Not analysing the evidence you use results in your writing being too descriptive, and not analytical (See *Chapter 5* for more information).

What your tutors say	What they mean
'How is this relevant?'	This means that what you have written does not help you answer the assignment question. Remember, when writing an assignment you are being asked to answer a particular question or solve a specific problem. Effective planning helps to keep your assignment focused and relevant.
'Your paragraphs need further development'/ 'Paragraph structure'	This means that you have used paragraphs incorrectly. They are either too long, or too short. Each paragraph should be focused on one point or idea. Each paragraph should follow the same basic structure: • Topic sentence • Evidence and analysis • Concluding remark

These are only a few examples of common feedback comments you may receive on your assignments. If you receive comments or suggestions you do not understand, book an appointment with your tutor to clarify any queries you may have.

ACTIVITY 8.5: SUBMISSION CHECKLIST

Look back at your last few pieces of assignment feedback, note any recurring comments ('avoid contractions', 'reference needed', 'lack of structure', and so on). Use these recurring comments to create a bespoke and personalised submission checklist to aid editing and proofreading.

Keep tweaking and adapting your submission checklist as your skills develop, as well as in response to new assignment feedback. Take things out that you no longer need reminding about; add new things as they are mentioned by your tutors. This ensures your checklist develops at the same time as you do.

Compare your initial submission checklist to the one you have at the end of the year. This is a good way to see exactly how your skills have developed over time and the progress you have made.

8.6 Marking rubrics

Another method that tutors can use to offer feedback to students following assessment is by using a rubric. Rubrics are a type of matrix that help students and tutors understand a set of criteria or dimensions of quality for any given type of assessment. These are usually designed with a particular assessment in mind (essay, presentation) and offer both student and tutor a means to communicate the assessment expectations and how grade-related criteria need to be met by each student.

All of the grade types and values are listed in a table and show students where they will be marked along the continuum of desired standards (see *Table 8.1*). This usually starts

Table 8.1 *Example of part of a marking rubric*

90–100 (1st class)	Develops new knowledge or novel perspective going beyond the literature	Work produced could hardly be bettered when produced under parallel conditions
80–89 (1st class)	Extensive subject knowledge with detailed insight into and understanding of relevant theory	Sophisticated understanding of complexities of key theoretical models, concepts and arguments
70–79 (1st class)	Extensive, thorough coverage of topic, focused use of detail and examples	Excellent, very sound understanding of complexities of key theoretical models, concepts and arguments
60–69 (upper second)	Breadth and depth of coverage, accurate and relevant in detail and example	Clear, sound understanding of subject matter, theory, issues and debate
50–59 (lower second)	Content generally relevant and accurate, most central issues identified; basic knowledge sound but may be patchy	Reasonable level of understanding of subject matter, theory and ideas; main issues satisfactorily understood
40–49 (third class)	Fairly basic knowledge, limited consistency of depth and accuracy of detail; not all aspects addressed, some omissions	Partial understanding of subject matter, core concepts and relevant issues; basic reference to theory
30–39 (Fail)	Contains very slight detail; content may be thin or irrelevant; issues poorly identified	Very little understanding of subject matter, ideas and issues; may be issue of misreading/misinterpretation of question
20–29 (Fail)	Little relevance of content; unacceptably weak or inaccurate knowledge base	Significant weaknesses and gaps in understanding of subject matter, ideas and issues; misunderstanding of question
10–19 (Fail)	Knowledge base extremely weak; content almost entirely irrelevant or erroneous	Devoid of understanding of subject matter, ideas and issues
0–9 (Fail)	Material not relevant or correct; no evidence of knowledge	No relevant understanding evident; response to question virtually nil

with the highest possible level of achievement in the left column and moves along the continuum to the far right column, which would denote the least-desirable standard. Each of the descriptions of the possible levels of attainment are written in sufficient detail to enable them to be useful for judgement of progress toward the module learning outcomes.

HELPFUL HINT

Use rubrics to provide another opportunity for dialogue between you and your tutor. If tutors do not offer the rubric to you alongside the assessment brief, ask whether this framework for assessment can be given in advance of your summative assessment to give you a better idea of what is expected of you. Rubrics are another opportunity for you to access a snapshot of information about your performance.

8.7 What to do after you receive feedback

- Store, download and save your feedback as soon as you get it. Keep your saved feedback in an easily identifiable location (either physically or electronically).
- Do not just check the overall grade, read all of your tutor's comments. Note down both the positives and the negatives.
- Look for recurring comments or themes. Add these to your submission checklist.
- Create action plans.
- If you need extra guidance and clarity, make an appointment to discuss the feedback with your tutor.

HELPFUL HINT

If you are disappointed with your mark and feedback, be kind to yourself. Have a bubble bath, a pint with friends, walk the dog, or do whatever it is you do to unwind. Then give yourself a day or two to reflect before making an appointment to see your tutor and/or study skills advisor.

8.8 Conclusion

This chapter has discussed the importance of maintaining a positive and proactive attitude to using feedback to aid your academic and personal development. Using feedback effectively allows you to plan your own progress, improve your grades, stay motivated and build resilience. Utilising the methods outlined above will enable you to become a resilient and independent learner, capable of self-assessment and self-regulation, all of which are key elements of lifelong learning.

SUMMARY

Four key points to take away from *Chapter 8*:
- ☑ Learning from your feedback can greatly improve your study skills.
- ☑ Obtaining feedback while writing your assignment can help you stay focused on your work.
- ☑ Feedback can be used to build resilience and lifelong learning skills.
- ☑ Giving and receiving feedback is an important employability skill.

Quiz

1. What is the purpose of feedback?

2. How does feedback benefit your education?

3. What do we mean by the term *feed-forward*?

4. How will building effective strategies to deal with negative and positive feedback affect your future career?

5. What does SMART stand for?

6. What can you do to make the most out of feedback?

7. What does the feedback comment 'Be more critical' mean?

8. What does the feedback comment 'Reference needed' mean?

REFERENCES

Boud, D. (2000) Sustainable assessment: rethinking assessment for the learning society. *Studies in Continuing Education*, 22(2), 151–67.

Butters, C., Kerfoot, S., Murphy, P. and Williams, A. (2013) 'I am just so delighted – now I know I can do it!' – How collaboration between nurse lecturers and academic skills tutors promotes students' confidence. *Journal of Learning Development in Higher Education*, No. 6. Retrieved from https://journal.aldinhe.ac.uk/index.php/jldhe/article/view/207 (last accessed 9 September 2019).

Duckworth, A. (2016) *Grit: the power of passion and perseverance*. Scribner.

Dweck, C. (2006) *Mindset: changing the way you think to fulfil your potential*. Random House.

Fry, H., Ketteridge, S., and Marshall, S. (2009) Understanding student learning. In Fry, H., Ketteridge, S. and Marshall, S. (eds) *A Handbook for Teaching and Learning in Higher Education: enhancing academic practice*, 3rd edition. Routledge.

Hounsell, D. (2004) 'Reinventing feedback for the contemporary Scottish university'. Paper presented at Quality Enhancement Workshop on 'Improving feedback to students', University of Glasgow, 4 June.

Mortiboys, A. (2005) *Teaching with Emotional Intelligence*. Routledge.

Nicol, D.J. (2010) From monologue to dialogue: improving written feedback processes in mass higher education. *Assessment & Evaluation in Higher Education*, 35(5), 501–17.

Nicol, D.J. and Macfarlane-Dick, D. (2006) Formative assessment and self-regulated learning: a model and seven principles of good feedback practice. *Studies in Higher Education*, 31(2), 199–218.

Pintrich, R.P. and Zusho, A. (2002) Student motivation and self-regulated learning in the college classroom. In Smart, J.C. and Tierney, W.G. (eds), *Higher Education: handbook of theory and research*, Volume XVII (pp. 55–128). Agathon Press.

Schön, D. (1987) *Educating the Reflective Practitioner: toward a new design for teaching and learning in the professions*. Jossey-Bass.

Chapter 9
Reflective writing skills

Marjorie Ghisoni

LEARNING OUTCOMES

When you have completed this chapter you should be able to:

9.1   Understand the process of reflection and reflective writing

9.2   Use reflective writing to improve your study skills and your care practice

9.3   Understand how reflective writing can benefit your lifelong learning and improve employability.

9.1 Introduction

Reflective writing as a skill has become an important part of professional practice and lifelong learning, as it can not only demonstrate knowledge development but can also be applied to individual practice as evidence of competent and compassionate care (Benner *et al.*, 2008). Reflective writing practice will also help you to develop your critical thinking skills so that your practice is evidence-based and up to date. See *Chapter 5* for more details about developing your critical thinking skills.

Research now shows that reflective writing can make a huge difference to the quality of care provided and to the health and well-being of people who need it (Royal College of Psychiatrists, 2015). Reflective writing helps us to develop compassionate care because it requires the practitioner to be aware of their own behaviour, the behaviour of the person they are working with and any conflicts or similarities between the two (Ghisoni, 2016).

This chapter will explore how reflective writing can help the student to become more resilient by developing their self-awareness and to be more person-centred when delivering health and social care. It will also look at outcomes for self-compassion, resilience and applying your knowledge to your everyday practice.

Developing academic writing skills in this area of practice will also enable practitioners to develop their confidence in providing good-quality care and being able to document how they have done it, thus demonstrating their employability to their managers and mentors, who might want to see evidence of professionalism and accountability. Developing your professional accountability skills will be explored further in *Chapter 12*.

Finally, reflective writing is now a requirement of some professional revalidation processes and can be developed into a lifelong learning skill. As you work through this chapter you will have the opportunity to practise reflective writing and to take some time to reflect on the way you develop the process of writing reflectively.

9.2 Models of reflective practice

Reflective practice is a state of mind, an ongoing attitude to life and work, the pearl grit in the oyster of practice and education; danger lies in it being a separate curriculum element with a set of exercises.

Bolton and Delderfield (2018, p. 1)

When learning about reflective practice and writing it can be useful to read around some theoretical models of reflection. You may not need to follow these models all of the time, but they can help you to develop your own model that will help you to practise reflective writing on a regular basis. Bolton and Delderfield (2018) argue that some models can restrict a person from reflecting upon their practice if they become prescriptive.

However, models of reflective practice can help us to get into the habit of writing reflectively and can be very useful at first. They can also help us to overcome obstacles to our reflective writing if we are struggling to identify areas of practice to reflect upon. Models of reflection might help people to reach a level of critical reflection that they would not be able to do by themselves. Most models will ask you to record your feelings because these can influence what you were thinking at the time of the event and how you might have reacted. Reflective writing should not just be used when something has gone wrong, because it can also help us to identify our skills in providing good care that we can share with others. Whichever model you use, the most important thing to remember is: what have I learnt from this?

Many models have developed from Kolb's adult learning cycle (*Figure 9.1*), which is a model of experiential learning that treats reflection as an integral part of learning (Kolb, 1984).

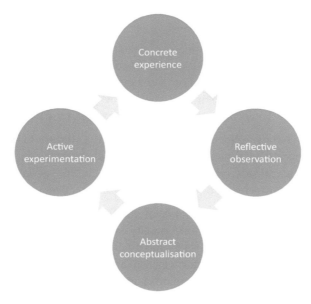

Figure 9.1 *Kolb's adult learning cycle.*

Stage 1:   Concrete experience

What was happening at the time, who were the actors and what did they do or say? This stage can be difficult to define and can prevent some people moving on to the next stage in the process. It is important here to focus on the *facts* of what happened, not how you felt during the event, as this can be identified and discussed in the next stage.

Stage 2:   Reflective observation

How did this make you feel, what was your initial reaction to the event? This is a good opportunity to separate out your feelings from the actual event. It can also help you to become more aware of your emotions and how they might influence your practice. It is not a bad thing to be emotional as it is a natural human response after all, and it can help you to define your compassion outcomes and skills.

Stage 3:   Abstract conceptualisation

What could have contributed to the event and what were the possible causes of the event happening? Here we move away from our emotions again to establish more facts. This helps us to identify triggers to an event that could, once identified, be managed differently next time if needed. It might also help us to identify what skills and behaviours were used to create a good outcome for the person involved.

Stage 4:   Active experimentation

After considering the above, what might you change, now that you know more and have reflected upon what happened? What can you do differently to improve the outcome of this event, should it happen again and what skills do you need to improve your practice? Some critics of reflective practice suggest that without this change taking place in our thinking, reflective writing and practice can be a useless exercise.

The four aspects of reflective writing or practice outlined below have since been developed by reflective writing theorists, but they all focus upon the learning that has taken place. One simple model is Oelofsen's three-step reflective cycle (Oelofsen, 2012), as shown in *Figure 9.2*.

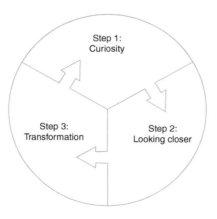

Figure 9.2 *Oelofsen's three-step reflective cycle.*

Step 1: Curiosity

As with Kolb's learning cycle, this step involves looking at the facts, but also noticing things, asking questions of yourself and questioning your assumptions.

Step 2: Looking closer

In this step, the practitioner zooms in on experiences and tries to make sense of events and feelings and put them into words.

Step 3: Transformation

This step is the key to making positive change. It involves using the observations from step 1 and the insights from step 2 to improve practice.

ACTIVITY 9.1

Read the scenario below and reflect upon how you could use your skills to help Jodie identify areas of her life to focus upon.

Jodie was a busy mum, wife and support worker who felt like she was always running around after everyone else and did not have a lot of time for herself. She decided to keep a diary of everything that happened in the day, just so she did not forget anything. One day she wrote about an event that puzzled her. It was about Eric, an older person she was looking after who was becoming very angry with her and she was not used to him being this way. Jodie did not know what had made Eric angry and thought that she needed to learn more about communicating with older people to understand what had happened.

Questions Jodie might ask of herself to reflect upon:
- Why did Eric get angry when he was usually very nice to her?
- How did Jodie feel when Eric was being angry towards her?
- What might make an older person angry when they are usually very nice?

Using Oelofsen's three-step model, Jodie might come up with the following reflection.

Step 1: Curiosity

Eric suddenly became angry and Jodie observed that this was unusual behaviour for him. She asked herself why he might have become angry so unexpectedly, and she also worried that she might have hurt him or said the wrong thing. Jodie felt upset that she might have caused Eric to become angry.

Step 2: Looking closer

Thinking about the episode more deeply was a good opportunity for Jodie to separate her feelings from the actual event. She began to think about what might have caused Eric to become angry. She realised she had been very busy that day and had not had time to talk to other carers about how Eric had been the day before. He might already have been in pain when she went to help him, or he might have been depressed about the illness affecting his life. Psychological support is an important part of Jodie's role but she may have not provided it very well that day because she was so busy.

Step 3: Transformation

After reflecting on the event, Jodie resolved to try to find time to talk to Eric's other carers before seeing him again. She decided that next time she might want to take more time with Eric if possible and ask him how he was feeling, demonstrating her compassion skills. Jodie also wanted to read more around psychological support and how she could develop her skills in providing it.

9.3 Should we follow our gut instinct?

People who write about professional development and reflective practice talk about 'perceptual acuity' (Benner *et al.*, 2008) or 'tacit' knowledge which in everyday language could be translated into our gut instinct. As we develop as professionals we are taught not to rely on our gut instinct but to use the evidence-based literature to support our practice. In reality we should do both. Schön (1983, cited in Smith, 2011) suggests that health and social care practice is not as clear-cut as we would like it to be or indeed as we would read in books such as this one. Instead, he argues that practice is messy and it does not fall into neat categories for us to work in. Developing our reflective practice can help us to sort out the messy reality of practice and to identify where we might need to improve. Using a model of reflection such as the ones outlined above can help us to develop our reflective thinking and writing skills so that it becomes a natural part of our everyday life.

In health and social care we are often presented with situations where we immediately think that something is not right; this is what most of us will be familiar with as our gut instinct. When we find ourselves in these situations our next thought tends to be, what we will do about it? Consider the following replies that we might give to ourselves:

a. Pretend you never saw/heard it.
b. Move closer to find out more.
c. Go and tell someone.
d. Go and think about it for a day or two before doing anything.

We might want to do all of the above, but we should also consider how our response will affect the situation – our first consideration as health and social care practitioners, under our professional codes, should always be to do no harm.

> ### ACTIVITY 9.2: READ THE FOLLOWING SCENARIO AND CONSIDER THE QUESTIONS BELOW
>
>
> *You have been asked to help Mrs Jones with preparing and eating a midday meal. You know that it is important for people to have a healthy diet and so you agree happily to help Mrs Jones. You have been studying healthy foods in your lectures and you want to put your new-found knowledge to the test. You have taken a great deal of time talking with Mrs Jones, finding out her favourite foods and making sure she had them on her shopping list so that you can now show her how to prepare and eat them.*

The cooking session goes very well and you feel like you are getting on really well with Mrs Jones. You leave Mrs Jones to eat her meal at the table while you clear up the pots and pans. You notice that Mrs Jones is coughing a lot and then she starts to choke on her food. You turn around to help her and offer to cut it up smaller so that it is easier to eat. Mrs Jones then enjoys the rest of her meal.

Upon reflection, you could say that it all went well at the time but there were a few things that may have triggered your gut instinct. All of the above options in this situation could be applied, but the scenario suggests that only option (b) was selected. When we use reflective practice we can consider all of the options to our gut reactions above, and reflect upon how we would respond in this situation in the future. Many of the theories around reflective practice focus upon what we did at the time (reflection *in* action) or afterwards (reflection *on* action), and while some people dispute how useful reflection actually is, it is still important to be aware of how it can help you to develop your gut instinct in practice so that you are practising safely. In reflective practice this is how we develop our knowledge and skills to address situations in practice better. Some of the situations you might now be considering reflecting on are:

1. Mrs Jones had told you what she liked to eat, but you had not asked her if there were any foods she found difficult to eat.
2. Mrs Jones appears to have a problem with swallowing, which may need to be checked out and advice sought on how this can be helped.
3. If Mrs Jones is struggling to eat healthily, her swallowing problems might be the reason why.
4. Mrs Jones is at risk of choking at home on her own if no one is around to help her.

The above simple scenario demonstrates how lifelong learning helps us to improve our reflective practice skills so that we can always be sure of using up-to-date knowledge and skills to practise safely. Reflective practice is very important to help us manage risk and to help the people that we care for to manage their own risk positively. Mrs Jones could still eat her favourite foods, but with advice from other professionals such as a dietician or a swallow assessment nurse, you have made sure that Mrs Jones is getting the best possible care and your gut instinct has been supported with up-to-date, evidence-based practice.

9.4 Keeping a reflective journal

Keeping a reflective journal is a useful tool in the reflective practitioner's kit. When studying for a course in healthcare there are many demands placed upon students to meet deadlines, while many students might also be working in a part-time job or looking after a busy family. This is where keeping a reflective journal can help you to prioritise what you need to do and put off those things that can wait.

Many of us enjoy studying already, which is why we want to develop ourselves through study and learning. However, if we do not learn how to learn, then much of what we do learn will become lost in our busy working and personal lives. Making time to reflect every day is important to help recognise where and how we learn, which can help us to develop further so that we can demonstrate safe and effective practice in our work.

Consider the following scenario and reflect upon what you can learn from it.

SCENARIO 9.1

A reflective journal entry by a healthcare student using Kolb's experiential learning model.

Concrete experience: I have an assignment deadline to meet and I am not sure if I am going to be able to do it. It is due in at the end of the month and my children have been off school with sickness just when I thought I was going to have time to finish it off.

Abstract reflection: I don't like to rush my assignments, but this one is not going to be as good as my other ones. I don't know what I can do to change this and I know I am going to fail!

Abstract conceptualisation: if I had gone to my tutorials on time and met my deadlines I would be better prepared. Maybe next time I need to think about keeping a diary of all of my deadlines so I can allow for things like this happening. I might also need to ask student support for some help with my study skills so I can be more organised. I could also ask for an extension to my assignment from the module tutor.

Active experimentation: contact the student support for help with managing my assignments and contact the module tutor for an extension to the submission deadline.

This student begins in panic mode and although they are usually well organised, they had not expected the children to be ill at the same time their assignment was due in. The above scenario demonstrates how the student became more resilient by reflecting upon the situation. The situation that this student finds themselves in can be changed a little, but in planning for the next assignment the student can develop their resilience to this stressful event better.

Examples of how the student might plan to change how they write their assignments in future are as follows:

- Regular contact with the tutor
- Write an assignment plan
- Use a calendar or diary to help keep themselves on track
- Join a journal group to discuss ideas
- Ask other students for help
- Find out what support systems are available in the university/college/school.

Why not add a few more of your own here?

 IMPROVING RESILIENCE, LIFELONG LEARNING AND EMPLOYABILITY

Reflective writing using models and frameworks such as those outlined above enables us to develop our resilience to the everyday events that can build up in our lives and cause stress and illness.

9.5 Developing reflective resilience in our everyday practice

Resilience is the way in which we develop skills and support to help us cope with a situation that is becoming stressful. While stress is difficult to define because it means different things to different people, resilience is not so difficult to define.

HELPFUL HINT

The resilience of an elastic band!

Think of an elastic band and how it is resilient to stretching. It always bounces back to its original shape. But if you stretch it too far, it will break. We may all think we have good coping skills around stressful events, but it only takes one extra stressor to tip us over the edge into panic mode. In using reflection to help us build up our resilience we can make it stronger and more prepared for the next stressful event that will come along. Why not wear an elastic band on your wrist to remind you how flexible you need to be to stay resilient?

ACTIVITY 9.3: BUILDING RESILIENCE

Make a note here of how many different ways you make time to reflect on your life.

You might have already explored your own resilience in *Chapter 1* and how you can develop it further through activities such as mindfulness or meditation, but for many people there might be other ways that help them better. Going for a long walk or doing some sporting activity can give us space to reflect, when sitting in front of a computer might not. The important thing to remember about reflective practice is finding a space where there are few distractions so that you can focus and if you are reflecting with another person or supervisor, where you can talk in privacy.

9.6 Reflective writing, self-compassion and student resilience

Using reflection as a way to build resilience is also a way to develop compassion for yourself. We often talk about a skill that we develop to help others, but if we cannot help ourselves first then we will probably not be very good at helping other people. This is something that is not taught very well in education settings, but many universities and colleges are now becoming more aware of how student self-compassion or resilience can affect their studies, their lives, their relationships and their individual success. Most education services are now providing student support around financial, physical, spiritual and mental health to help students cope with the demands of everyday life. If you think you might be experiencing a problem with your studies it is important to reflect upon the problem and then share it.

To explore student resilience in more depth visit the student resilience toolkit website produced by The Student Services Organisation: www.amosshe.org.uk. When considering or reflecting upon your own resilience remember the 5Rs that were discussed in *Chapter 1*:
Rest – am I getting enough rest so I can concentrate/reflect more?
Reflect – am I reflecting regularly?
Relax – am I finding time to do the things that make me happy?
Replenish – am I eating good food and avoiding harmful substances as much as possible?
Respire – am I making sure I am breathing properly each day?

The above five ways to develop your resilience as a student will help you to reflect and manage any risks that you might be not coping with very well. I have developed this checklist into a RISK (Resilience in Self Knowledge) score as a special page on my blogsite that can be used to check in and practise your reflection skills whenever you need to: https://drmarjorieghisoni.edublogs.org

9.6.1 Learning from our mistakes

As we are human beings and make mistakes, we can sometimes make people more dependent upon us when we should be helping them to become more independent. We might do this by becoming protective of the person or by not giving them the correct information to help themselves. This is clearly not our original intention, and we might be upset to find that we have not helped the person or family. However, without finding out this information we might only be doing more harm, which was never our intention in the first place. Reflective writing can include your own experiences and feelings, and this will develop your self-compassion. Reflection is a way of developing our skills and knowledge of legal and ethical practice and may begin an in-depth analysis of our own values and beliefs.

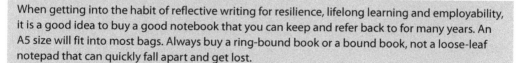

HELPFUL HINT ✔

When getting into the habit of reflective writing for resilience, lifelong learning and employability, it is a good idea to buy a good notebook that you can keep and refer back to for many years. An A5 size will fit into most bags. Always buy a ring-bound book or a bound book, not a loose-leaf notepad that can quickly fall apart and get lost.

Always write the full reference to anything you have read at the top of the page so it is easy to find and always record page numbers for direct quotations, so you do not have to go looking for them just before your assignment submission deadline is due.

9.7 Reflective writing and lifelong learning

As you can see from Kolb's experiential learning model and Oelofsen's three-step reflective cycle, reflective practice is continuous as your learning develops. The more you learn, the more you want to try out your new learning to improve your practice and ultimately to be more effective in the workplace. Reflective practice has developed from the field of education as people began to wonder how we learn best. This has led to research over many years to identify key components of reflective practice. It is not just about looking in the mirror at our practice, but it is more about stopping as we walk past the mirror to check that we are doing it right. It is also important to write about your reflective practice so that you can look back over time to see how your learning has developed. Many professional bodies now require us to do this as part of our professional registration. Some of the questions that might arise in reflective practice are:

- Why did I do that in that way?
- How do I know that that is the best way to do it?
- What can I do or change to make my practice better?

When we learn about things in our everyday lives we do not always recognise the learning that has taken place. The quote from Bolton and Delderfield (2018) in *Section 9.2* reminds us that reflective writing should not be a separate part of your study, but should be an integral part of everything that you do. Reflective practice needs to be developed in our daily lives so that it becomes a habit and a safe way to wind down at the end of a very busy day or week. As we have seen, reflective practice can help us to become more self-compassionate as we begin to recognise our own needs more and how they can be addressed. These needs include our lifelong learning needs, which enable us to continue to develop and carry out our work effectively. This is why it is important to reflect upon the day and to write down what you have learnt. Even if you revisit your reflective writing later, just having something to look at will help you to revisit your lifelong learning needs.

Reflective practice also helps us to become a more compassionate practitioner. As we reflect, we are also analysing events so that we can make sense of what took place. This involves separating out our feelings from the facts surrounding the event and identifying what knowledge we have or need to help people more effectively. If we were to become more reflective practitioners we should therefore become more compassionate practitioners. As we learn from our reflective practice, we are developing our lifelong learning skills and adding to those skills in a compassionate response to our practice with other human beings. Compassion is often talked about as a skill (Ghisoni, 2016) that should be evident in all health and social care practitioners, but unless we continually practise any skill we can become rusty and forget to use it. Reflective writing as a lifelong learning skill is an excellent way to keep all of your skills up to date by analysing how and when you have used them.

9.8 Professional requirements for reflective practice and lifelong learning

Reflective practice is also a requirement of many professional bodies and accompanies the requirement to keep your skills up to date, and it forms part of your lifelong learning or continuous professional development (CPD). For example, the Nursing and Midwifery Council (NMC, 2018) has developed a code of ethical practice that all nurses are expected to follow so that the people that they care for are kept safe. The NMC (2018, p. 4) states that all nurses need to be able to reflect upon their own practice:

You assess need and deliver or advise on treatment, or give help (including preventative or rehabilitative care) without too much delay and to the best of your abilities, on the basis of the best evidence available and best practice. You communicate effectively, keeping clear and accurate records and sharing skills, knowledge and experience where appropriate. You reflect and act on any feedback you receive to improve your practice.

This code has recently been updated to include Associate Practitioners in England. All nurses and associate practitioners are required to register with the NMC and the public can check that people are up-to-date in their practice. In addition, all registered nurses have to revalidate every three years, and this process includes preparing five written reflective accounts of:

- An instance of your continuous professional development, and/or
- A piece of practice-related feedback you have received, and/or
- An event or experience in your own professional practice.

All these accounts must also describe how they relate to the NMC Code. You can visit the advice and guidelines on the NMC website here: www.nmc.org.uk

Other health and social care professionals have similar codes of practice like this one from the Social Care Services for Wales (2017, p. 15; see website for more information: www.socialcare.wales).

You must be accountable for the quality of your work and take responsibility for maintaining and developing knowledge and skills.

and the Royal College of Occupational Therapists (RCOT, 2015, p. 41) Code of Ethics and Professional Conduct:

Critical reflective thinking underpins the bringing together of different ideas and application of all professional development activities to the benefit of your service user/s, your service and yourself. You will be able to demonstrate how you have developed your critically reflective thinking skills throughout your professional journey.

See the RCOT(2015) website for more information: www.rcot.co.uk

Developing our individual reflective practice not only helps us to develop our own individual resilience through our writing and communication skills but also demonstrates our professional development and lifelong learning, as required by many of our professional bodies. Developing our skills in professional practice and how these fit with professional codes is discussed more in *Chapter 13*. Reflective practice is outlined within this chapter as an important part of our professional development as it can help us learn from our experiences and mistakes and can also help us to develop our skills in resilience using the 5Rs discussed in *Chapter 1*. Developing resilience and lifelong learning skills through reflection can also help us by default to develop our employability skills, making that dreamed-for job more likely to become a reality.

9.9 **Reflective writing for employability**

Employability often depends on the skills and knowledge that you have and the skills and knowledge that employers need. This becomes more evident when you start to apply for jobs in your professional field. However, it is worth considering here what skills and knowledge you might need to be more attractive to future employers. Fill in the boxes in *Activity 9.4* as you learn about different health and social care professions to help you identify the different skills and knowledge that are required of different professional groups.

ACTIVITY 9.4

Professional field	Skills	Knowledge	Reflective points
Each field will be different but some skills and knowledge may be shared	*e.g. communication*	*e.g. anatomy*	*What do you think are the most important skills and knowledge?*
Nursing	Personal care	Health and healing	
Social work			
Radiography			
Occupational therapy			
Physiotherapy			
Speech therapy			
Counselling			
Medical care			
Associate practitioners			

9.9.1 Graduateness and employability

As we become more aware of different professional groups that we may be working with in the future, we also become more aware of the skills that all professionals will share in their working lives. Sometimes it is difficult when working in busy practice areas to see beyond the blurring of professional boundaries, which is why it is important to reflect upon how we can all work together more effectively. Knowing the skills and knowledge of other professionals will help you to provide the best care for the people you are working with.

When we consider preparation for employment after leaving university, we talk about how prepared students are by their 'graduateness': this means looking at how equipped students are to face the world of full-time professional responsibility, and this can be a difficult time in your academic career. In *Chapter 12* we discuss graduateness further in relation to employability and how the skills that you develop during your time as a student can be transferable to the working environment. In order to develop those employability skills as you develop your knowledge and study skills, you can use reflection and reflective practice as a tool to keep a check on which skills you might need to develop more. Here are some tips about what graduateness for employability means:

- Acting professionally at all times and reflecting upon and referring to your code of practice
- Acting legally and ethically at all times and reflecting upon and referring to your health and social care law, codes of practice and policy
- Continuing to develop your critical thinking skills and reflective writing to make sure every person you care for can get access to the best evidence-based care available
- Continuing to support your peers and mentors with the challenges facing health and social care services in the future through reflection and peer support
- Reflecting continually on your own practice and developmental needs and thinking and talking about further study after graduating.

It can be very reassuring to know that all professionals will need to be able to demonstrate their knowledge and skills in practice. One way we can all do this is by using reflective practice more and developing these skills with our peers and in our individual professional lives. Reflective practice is not an add-on skill when we have time to do it, which is often what you will see in practice. This is not being self-compassionate, and in some situations can lead to poor practice and ineffective outcomes. If your prospective employer knows that you are a reflective practitioner they will be more likely to employ you knowing that you are also a safe and reflective practitioner.

9.10 **Conclusion**

Skills for reflective writing are often personal and unique, but there are some ways that you can develop your reflective writing skills. This chapter has explored how reflective writing can help us to learn continuously through lifelong learning and to develop our skills of resilience in our professional and personal lives. Reflective writing is perhaps most helpful when we are seeking employability within an environment that is caring and compassionate. Demonstrating reflective writing skills to our prospective employers and our peers also demonstrates that we have good resilience skills that we can use to develop our professional practice in the workplace.

SUMMARY

Four key points to take away from *Chapter 9*:
- ☑ Reflection can help you to become more aware of your own needs and skills.
- ☑ Resilience and self-compassion can help you to become more reflective in your everyday life.
- ☑ Reflective practice helps you to improve your skills and knowledge in your practice.
- ☑ Reflective practice improves the quality of your writing as it demonstrates your knowledge and practice development.

Quiz

1. Whose model of reflection was one of the first to be used in education?
2. What type of writing helps us to develop compassionate care?
3. What is another term for gut instinct?
4. What is the term for reflecting while in practice?
5. What is the term for reflecting about practice?

REFERENCES

Benner, P., Hughes, R.G. and Sutphen, M. (2008) Clinical reasoning, decisionmaking and action: thinking critically and clinically. In Hughes, R.G. (ed.) *Patient Safety and Quality: an evidence-based handbook for nurses*. Agency for Healthcare Research.

Bolton, G. and Delderfield, R. (2018) *Reflective Practice: writing and professional development*, 5th edition. Sage.

Ghisoni, M. (2016) The components of compassion. In Hewison, A. and Sawbridge, Y. (eds) *Compassion in Nursing: theory, evidence and practice*. Oxford University Press.

Kolb, D.A. (1984) *Experiential Learning: experience as the source of learning and development*. Prentice Hall.

Nursing and Midwifery Council (2018) *The Code: professional standards of practice and behaviour for nurses, midwives and nursing associates*. NMC.

Oelofsen, N. (2012) *Developing Reflective Practice: a guide for students and practitioners of health and social care*. Lantern Publishing.

Royal College of Psychiatrists (2015) *Compassion in Care: ten things you can do to make a difference*. The Royal College of Psychiatrists. Faculty Report GAP/02.

Smith, M.K. (2011) Donald Schön: learning, reflection and change. *The Encyclopedia of Informal Education*. Available at: www.infed.org/thinkers/et-schon.htm (accessed 9 September 2019).

Chapter 10
Skills for teamworking

Liz Lefroy

LEARNING OUTCOMES

When you have completed this chapter you should be able to:

10.1 Understand how to become an effective member of a team

10.2 Understand why teamworking is important for safe practice

10.3 Understand your role in a team

10.4 Work towards team goals

10.5 Communicate effectively with other members of a team

10.6 Sustain the ability to work in teams throughout your career.

10.1 Introduction

Teams are everywhere. You may already belong to several: a sports team, the committee which organises a student society, a choir. Becoming a professional in the field of health and social care requires attention to ideas of teamwork, because in the future your ability to work with others will be among the key skills sought by prospective employers. The good news is that the learning can start now: with your engagement with fellow students, and with your colleagues during work experience placements. The lecture room itself provides many opportunities for practising teamwork skills. Just as an ability to study alone is essential, learning with others can bring benefits and opportunities as students can share ideas, gain extra perspectives and stimulate one another's thinking.

The learning outcomes of the chapter focus on the knowledge underpinning the key question: *What are the skills needed for effective teamworking in health and social care contexts?* An ability to answer this question will give you a blueprint to apply to any team in which you are placed: from the small group working together on classroom tasks to the multidisciplinary team in which you secure a job in your first year in practice. This focus on identification of skills is made because effective teamworking, at its most straightforward, is characterised by a good match between a team's aims and its outcomes.

10.2 **What is a team?**

Teams are formed for two main reasons – either when the quantity of work is too great for one person or when the task that needs to be completed requires a diversity of specialisms. Many teams in which you are likely to work are formed from a combination of these *quantity* and *diversity* needs. Teams can increase individuals' ability to work effectively and safely.

ACTIVITY 10.1

Do you consider the following to be teams?
A – You and your closest course colleagues
B – Your whole year group
C – Everyone involved in your degree programme

In social care and health professions, the notion of a team is flexible and contextual. In its most literal sense, it is a group of people assigned a specific task, usually headed by a leader. West *et al.* (1998) identify that a team has three characteristics:

- A clear organisational identity
- A shared purpose
- Members whose roles are interlinked.

All the examples in *Activity 10.1* could be argued to have features of a team – in example A, you share a clear identity and goal with fellow students on the same course. Example C comes closer still to meeting the characteristics of a team with lecturers, administrators, fellow students, the professional regulatory body, practitioners and individuals who use services, all contributing through their particular roles to the end goal of training future health and social care professionals.

A team is not formed simply by collecting people together. Jelphs *et al.* (2016, p. 7), referring to the work of Dawson *et al.* (2009), differentiate between 'pseudo' teams and 'real' teams. The former are groups arranged in a structure to achieve a task but they do not achieve it. In contrast, a real team is one in which each member understands the team's objectives and works consistently towards them. The way a team is labelled (for example, *Initial Assessment Team*) helps both those working within it and those receiving its services to understand their objectives. Some team terminology needs further explanation. *Table 10.1* is a rough guide to the phrases you might come across as you progress through your education. You can use the table to identify which of these terms applies to the teams you encounter.

The terms multidisciplinary and interdisciplinary are often used interchangeably, but Fawcett (2013, p. 376) makes the following distinction:

Multidisciplinary refers to knowledge that is drawn from diverse disciplines but the research questions and methods stay within the distinct boundaries of each discipline.
Interdisciplinary research involves an integrative and reciprocally interactive approach.

Table 10.1 *Team terminology*

Type of team	Practitioners	Features	Your example
Multiprofessional team	All from the same professional discipline	Colleagues within the same profession but probably having different specialisms	
Multidisciplinary team	From two or more different professions	Practitioners are chosen to meet the variety of needs of the individuals they seek to support, and divide up tasks according to disciplines	
Multi-agency team	From two or more different agencies	Team members may have different employers, e.g. NHS and Local Authority	
Interdisciplinary team	From two or more different professions	Works collaboratively towards goals, rather than as individual practitioners	

In clinical settings, surgical teams have traditionally been interdisciplinary. In *Scenario 10.1*, a former Theatre Nurse, someone who now supports the education of social workers and nurses from the point of view of someone who uses services, describes her experience of teamwork during life-saving operations.

SCENARIO 10.1: INTERDISCIPLINARY TEAMWORK AND NURSING NARRATIVE

Ward ➡
    Recovery Nurse ➡
        Anaesthetic Team ➡
                Surgical Team
        Anaesthetic Team ⬅
    Recovery Nurse ⬅
Ward ⬅
            The handover of patient care for continuous support

My memories of working as a theatre nurse are very positive. There was a team for each stage of the surgical process, ensuring continuity of care for all patients from the time they left the ward, through surgery, to the point of return to the ward. The recovery team looked after the patient before and after surgery. The anaesthetic team took care of the patient immediately prior to surgery and stayed with the patient throughout, becoming part of the team during the surgical procedure. The surgical team consisted of the surgeon, the junior doctor, the scrubbed nurse, and the runners. An operation cannot occur without the full team being in place and all communication between the teams being completed.

The patient was the team leader even when unconscious. Everything revolved around his or her needs. The ultimate responsibility lay with the surgeon, but each team member was important and responsible for her/his duties. In the role of recovery nurse, I had to make sure all the documentation was in order and accurate before the operation could take place, while reassuring the patient and answering any last-minute questions. As the scrubbed nurse, I was the patient's advocate, also ensuring that all instruments, sharps and swabs were accounted for before and at the end of the operation. The anaesthetic team and the scrubbed nurse individually handed over the care of the patient back to the recovery nurse, who ensured that when the patient was handed back to the ward, she/he was conscious and comfortable.

No one had power over anyone else in the operating theatre. Outside, we might not have anything in common, but once inside and working together we were totally focused on the job and respected our interdependence. All communication was kept clear and pared down to the essentials – there was no chit chat.

We also had to be strong enough to challenge each other over anything. We needed to know our limitations, our weaknesses and strengths – you had to ask for help before you got to the point of needing it.

It was an honour to be part of the theatre team – you had to earn your place!

Eluned Plack, former Theatre Nurse

While not all team experiences have this intensity, this description exemplifies the principles of interdisciplinary working which can be applied in other situations: focus on the patient, clarity of goals, precise communication, accountability to the patient and each other.

Different professions have particular pathways to qualification, but understanding the focus of other disciplines is essential for safe practice in health and social care. Health and social work is regulated by professional bodies that stipulate national occupational standards like the example below.

> *Effective multi-disciplinary work is an essential component of social work: the information known to different agencies must be shared to identify those at risk, the skills of different professions must be coordinated to benefit those with complex requirements, the resources of different agencies must be pooled to maximise person centred outcomes*
>
> CCW, 2011, NOS 6

Individuals must be at the centre of provision and agencies must work collaboratively towards outcomes which may either be agreed together, or in some cases imposed because of risk to individuals' welfare. This poses challenges, not least because health and social care agencies have been set up with differing working structures and practices. For example, in his report following the death of Peter Connelly (Baby P), Lord Laming wrote that 'cooperative efforts are often first to suffer' when professionals are under pressure (Laming, 2009, para. 4.3).

Successive governments before and since this tragedy have sought to address issues of poor communication across professional boundaries by taking actions such as combining education and social services within single management structures. Whatever the structure, however, the potential for mis- or non-communication needs to be anticipated and proactive habits developed by those new to practice.

10.3 Teamwork in a time of change

In addition to working across professional boundaries as suggested above, contemporary teams often have multiple remits, and carry out many functions in virtual rather than actual space. In the health and social care sector, organisational restructuring, developments in information technology and environmental considerations are just as challenging. Services in health and social care have consequently evolved from a period of austerity, as Jelphs *et al.* (2016, p. 1) comment that 'government and non-government organisations alike are tasked with … doing more with fewer resources' and all this in a climate of higher expectations.

For many, the teams they have been used to working in have been reconfigured, with some team members being redeployed or losing their jobs. Changes in information technology, along with the sale of assets such as buildings, mean that teams can be expected to work remotely, no longer seeing each other daily. Legislation which seeks to respond to changes in demographics, such as an ageing population, also has specific impacts. Given these demands, students in health and social care professions will be facing situations which are challenging even to experienced professionals. Developing individual resilience, as discussed in *Chapter 1*, will help the student to recognise and develop individual knowledge and skills. One way in which this can be achieved is to identify the different roles in teams and where their skills might lie.

10.4 Team role theory

In the context of a workforce undergoing regular reorganisation, a theoretical basis for teamwork which is adaptable to different circumstances is essential. In the learning outcomes identified at the start of this chapter, *the ability to understand your role in a team* encompasses not only your growing awareness of your professional interests and strengths, but also the *way* in which you function within teams.

Belbin's (2018) highly influential Team Role Theory can help the developing practitioner to understand the anatomy of teams. He observed that there are typically nine roles that need to be fulfilled by one or more person within a team.

ACTIVITY 10.2

Imagine you are starting a practice placement next week. You have previously been employed for five years as a team leader within a residential home and are worried about how you are going to manage returning to a student role. How could an understanding of Belbin's team role theory contribute to reducing your anxiety?

Table 10.2 *The Team Role Theory of Meredith Belbin*

Shaper	This person is driven and wants to make progress towards goals quickly. She keeps a team focused and active.
Plant	This person is creative and has many ideas, which are not necessarily practical but can be turned into reality by the team.
Monitor Evaluator	This person questions what the group is doing. His questioning can prevent the team from making mistakes.
Completer Finisher	This person has an eye for detail, spotting gaps and errors. The Shaper and the Completer Finisher may irritate each other.
Implementer	This person can take a problem and work out how to solve it. Her practical approach may sometimes clash with the Plant's innovative ideas.
Resource Investigator	This person can help the team to solve its problems by networking outside the team.
Team Worker	This person helps to facilitate the interpersonal relationships within the team.
Coordinator	This person ensures that all members of the team have their say. He understands that listening to all views can result in better decisions.
Specialist	This person brings specialist knowledge to the team.

None of Belbin's team roles depends on rank or line management responsibility. A student can be effective as a Monitor Evaluator, for example: asking questions falls naturally into the remit of learning. You may bring a Specialist's knowledge to the team from your past role, especially if you have had intensive contact with individuals needing particular forms of support, or have been in receipt of services yourself.

As well as being sensitive to the need for team members with different characteristics, in order to be clear about your role you must understand the professional basis from which you practise. Who, for example, regulates your chosen profession? What is its code of ethics, its key roles? This professional identity may feel quite vague at present: comparing your emerging professional role with that of others brings greater clarity. If you are training to be a nurse, do you know how your role will differ from that of an occupational therapist? Use *Table 10.3* to build your understanding of each of the different professions, basing your answers on the country in which you are studying. The first line has been completed as an example.

10.5 The development of groups and teams

Jelphs *et al.*'s (2016) criticism of pseudo teams comes from evidence demonstrating that these teams are more likely to practise in unsafe ways. West and Lyubovnikova (2013, p. 138)

Table 10.3 *Index of different health and social care professions*

Profession title	Regulatory body	Code of ethics	Professional membership body	Documents describing key professional roles
Nurse (UK)	Nursing and Midwifery Council	The Code: professional standards of practice and behaviour for nurses, midwives and nursing associates	Royal College of Nursing	*Future Nurse: standards of proficiency for registered nurses* (NMC, 2018)
Occupational Therapist				
Social Worker				
Psychologist				
Dietician				
Approved Mental Health Practitioner				
Psychiatrist				
Your role (if not mentioned above)				

state that 'research consistently shows that it is common for team members to be unclear about exactly what the objectives of the team are, thereby making inter-dependent working more difficult'. Dawson *et al.* (2009, cited in Jelphs *et al.*, 2016) state that teams without clear goals make more mistakes, and have members who experience lower levels of well-being. In the learning outcomes identified at the start of this chapter, *the ability to understand and work towards the team's goals* is crucial to forming and sustaining real, goal-orientated teams.

As a student professional in health and social care, your understanding of a team's goals will be dependent on the complexity of those goals and how clearly they are expressed. The issue of leadership within teams in health and social care can be problematic, as West and Lyubovnikova (2013) found, with clear lines of responsibility not always present. Where leadership is strong, goals are well-defined and support for excellence and innovation was higher. You are unlikely to have strategic influence for a long while, but you have a part to play in any team in ensuring that you understand its goals.

IMPROVING RESILIENCE, LIFELONG LEARNING AND EMPLOYABILITY

Understanding a team's goals and your role in achieving those goals will help your employability when you come to apply for jobs.

In the case of teams located within organisations with statutory responsibilities, such as local authorities or the National Health Service, goals are often determined by legislation and policy. They could include working to very specific time limits, for example those relating to safeguarding children and adults. If you are placed in a team in the community – for example, within a charity, private company or social enterprise – goals may be broadly defined in a mission statement, with more precise goals being articulated in organisational policy, job descriptions and project aims. Koprowska (2010, p. 13) notes that 'the goals of voluntary organisations may have more in common with each other than those of statutory agencies working with the same user group'. *Activity 10.3* cites the impressive mission statement of Hafal, a third-sector organisation in Wales which is managed by people who have experience of serious mental illness and their families. In their Input–Output model of team effectiveness, West and Lyubovnikova's (2013) first requirement and measure of effectiveness is clarity about the team task.

ACTIVITY 10.3

Read the example below and then discuss with a fellow student what each of you understands by the term 'a better quality of life'.

Example – A mission statement

'Hafal is founded on the belief that people who have direct experience of mental illness know best how services can be delivered.

Providing support across the seven local health board areas of Wales, Hafal is dedicated to empowering people with serious mental illness and their families to:
1. Achieve a better quality of life
2. Fulfil their ambitions for recovery
3. Fight discrimination
4. Enjoy equal access to health and social care, housing, income, education, and employment.'

www.hafal.org/about

As a student practitioner, your understanding of the standards required for professional working needs to be developed in each new situation. Part of the skill is being prepared for the trajectory this learning will take. A useful theory when considering the development of teams is that of Tuckman (1965), who observed small groups going through a process of forming, storming, norming and performing (*Table 10.4*). Later, Tuckman and Jensen (1977) added a fifth stage: adjourning. While this theory was developed in the context of small groups rather than teams, the theoretical understanding is useful here.

At the forming stage, people get together and establish goals. In terms of the student experience, this could be a meeting prior to a work experience placement at which those involved record what it is the student aims to learn. To some extent, these goals are pre-determined by the requirements of the course, but the nuances, what this particular experience can teach this particular student, need to be made transparent.

Tuckman's (1965) research showed that the storming phase (the point at which initial pleasantries may be overtaken by irritations and disappointments about other team members) only occurred in approximately 50% of the groups studied – some moved straight to the third stage. If you do recognise a storming phase, however, it's reassuring to know that it is a common experience.

Norming is the stage at which the student begins to feel part of the group or team. She can start to perform tasks with increasing confidence, moving to the performing stage, during which the focus is on the achievement of goals. Placements inevitably come to an end, and adjourning is experienced, which may include emotions of anxiety and sadness or relief.

Table 10.4 *Tuckman's Model of Group Development in Health and Social Care*

Forming	Developing group resilience, e.g. identifying strengths and weaknesses	Developing group rules for employability, e.g. identifying workload/mission	Developing group rules for lifelong learning and development
Storming	Sharing group resilience skills	Sharing group employability skills	Sharing group knowledge
Norming	Developing individual resilience, e.g. identifying roles	Developing group activities for employability	Developing group knowledge and skills for lifelong learning
Performing	Using group resilience skills, e.g. caseloads	Using group employability skills, e.g. workload	Using group knowledge and skills
Adjourning	Completing resilience tasks	Completing employability tasks	Completing shared learning and skill development

10.6 Communication and sustainable teamwork

The ability to communicate effectively with other team members is identified in the learning outcomes for this chapter as crucial to sustainable teamwork. Learning in groups and working in teams crucially involves listening to others. Koprowska (2010, p. 79) remarks that 'listening attentively conveys interest and respect, and is an essential part of the turn-taking that characterises human interaction'. Active listening incorporates skills such as nodding to show understanding, giving eye contact, smiling and avoiding distracting others by fidgeting.

ACTIVITY 10.4: ACTIVE LISTENING

How do you know when someone is listening to you? How do you like them to show this?

If you're listening actively, how would you demonstrate this when speaking with someone who:
- Has a visual impairment?
- Has a hearing impairment or is deaf?

A simple model of communication (*Figure 10.1*) demonstrates how easily a connection can be broken or distorted. Interference in the cycle of communication can take many forms: external pressures such as geographical separation or other resource issues, or intrinsic factors, such as use of professional jargon, inadequate understanding of common goals, or personal characteristics such as unreliability, or lack of confidence.

10.7 Dealing with conflict

The complex nature of interpersonal relationships makes conflict a predictable experience in teamworking. There are a number of reasons why conflict may occur, particularly in teams formed of people from different professions or disciplines.

10.7.1 Diversity

Jelphs *et al.* (2016, p. 58) comment that, while diversity can act as a strengthening factor, 'different professions may also have different perspectives of what good teamwork looks like' – 'essentially people see the world differently' (p. 74). Teams in which communication is poor do not fulfil their goals at best, and at worst operate in an atmosphere of exhaustion and can make serious errors. Students, while they may often feel relatively powerless, can

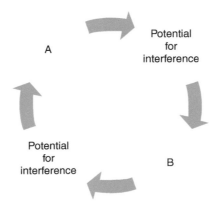

Figure 10.1 *A model of communication.*

nevertheless learn skills and practices that will ensure a better outcome in group or team situations.

10.7.2 Intrinsic factors

The intrinsic factors causing interference in communication can be addressed by individuals committed to teamworking. In *The Art of Social Work Practice*, Weinstein (2008, p. 133) states that it is 'important to come to any new inter-professional relationship … from an *"I'm ok, you're ok"'* (Harris, 1995) position. Perhaps unsurprisingly, the qualities valued by individuals who use services coincide with those which promote good communication: the same qualities of reliability, honesty and dependability. These are demonstrated in skills such as turning up on time, replying promptly to phone calls and emails, being clear about purpose, listening, and offering practical support rather than defensive responses when challenged.

10.7.3 Communication skills

Practising clear and timely communication skills, and noticing the positive effects that result, will help reinforce good practice in readiness for the workplace. Initially, learning about teamwork and effective communication may occur in classroom activities. *Case Example 10.3* describes the experience of a first-year student during a small group-work activity carried out as part of the social work degree on which I teach. The student was assigned to work in a small group of five to produce a presentation after six weeks. One of the group is a member of Outside In (Morris *et al.*, 2013), the focus group which is formed of people who have experienced using health and social care services, and who contribute this expertise to the degree in a variety of ways. This example illustrates the student's viewpoint of the interpersonal and communication skills used in teamwork.

CASE EXAMPLE 10.3: PRACTISING COMMUNICATION SKILLS

We began the assignment by introducing ourselves to each other and particularly to X, who is a member of Outside In. We set some ground rules to protect each other while working together with a basis of trust, amiability and respect. Beresford (2012) reports that service users identify their relationship with their social worker as of critical importance to them, with value placed on working together as opposed to 'us and them'. The findings from Beresford et al. (2006) suggest that when individuals and students work together in an educational setting this is on equal terms, which I felt our group dynamic reflected. During our group-work sessions we were able to fully appreciate the benefits of our teamwork and participation and it was evident that I fulfilled the role of 'Co-ordinator' in Belbin's Team Role Theory (2018). Here my own values emerged and helped to ensure that all members of the group's suggestions were heard.

Taking part in the group assignment was an advantageous experience as I was able to see the reality of how communications skills impact individuals and myself, by gaining immediate feedback.

Abbie Watkins, Year 1 Social Work Student

TEAM SKILLS   YOUR GOALS

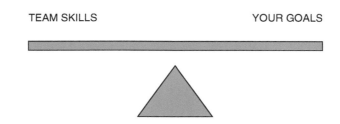

Figure 10.2 *Achieving balance.*

So, let's imagine you have reached the point at which you can demonstrate the ability to understand your role in a team, the ability to understand and work towards the team's goals and the ability to communicate effectively with other team members. How will you develop the ability to sustain all these activities throughout your career?

10.8 **Resilience**

Resilience, a key theme of this book, is important here, and other chapters will interact with this one, increasing your understanding of sustainable practice. Perhaps ironically within a chapter on teamworking, this last section is dedicated to the imperative to look after yourself. Self-care within the team setting is crucial, and an aspect of this relates to the subject of goals with which much of this chapter has been concerned. Specifically, rather than being at odds with a team's goals, a focus on your own goals is also essential. *Figure 10.2* uses the simple illustration of a see-saw as an *aide memoire* – you need to maintain balance between the aims of the team within which you study or work and your own professional goals. In their model of collaboration as a means for approaching conflict situations, Kilmann and Thomas (1977) argue that they are most readily resolved when equal priority is given by professionals to team and personal goals.

ACTIVITY 10.5: TEAM SKILLS: YOUR GOALS

- What are your goals for your professional career in the next five years?
- How do these goals relate to the goals of the team you last worked with?
- What will you do to achieve a better balance between your own goals and those of the team when you are next involved in working in a team?

10.9 **Conclusion**

This chapter has moved from a theoretical understanding of teams and teamwork through practical examples and exercises to a focus on the skills that individual practitioners will need to gain and sustain employment. To be part of a team which practises effectively and safely, you will need to develop a clear understanding of your professional aims and

objectives, alongside the ability to integrate team goals into every element of your practice. The first step in doing this in any new team environment is to ensure that you understand what those goals are, and if you are unsure, to persist in your quest to find out.

SUMMARY

Four key points to take away from *Chapter 10*:
- ☑ Working in teams is common practice in health and social care.
- ☑ Teamworking skills are important for effective service delivery.
- ☑ Learning how to work in a team is a good way to develop employability skills.
- ☑ Good team players want the best available service for people in their care.

Quiz

1. What are the three features which define a team, according to West *et al.* (1998)?

2. Name the four stages of Tuckman's original (1965) theory of the life cycle of groups and teams.

3. Which stage did Tuckman and Jensen add in 1977?

4. How does a multidisciplinary team differ from an interdisciplinary team?

5. What is the difference between a 'pseudo' team and a 'real' team?

REFERENCES AND FURTHER READING

Belbin, M. (2018) The Nine Belbin Team Roles. Retrieved from www.belbin.com/about/belbin-team-roles/ (accessed 9 September 2019).

Beresford, P. (2012) *What service users want from social workers*. Community Care. Retrieved from www.communitycare.co.uk/2012/04/27/what-service-users-want-from-social-workers/ (accessed 9 September 2019).

Beresford, P., Branfield, F., Taylor, J., Brennan, A., Satori, A., Lalani, M. and Wise, G. (2006) Working together for better social work education. *Social Work Education – The International Journey*, 25(4), 326–31.

Care Council for Wales (2011) *National Occupational Standards for Social Work*. Care Council for Wales.

Dawson, J.F., West, M.A. and Yan, X. (2009) Positive and negative effects of team working in health care: 'real' and 'pseudo' teams and their effect on healthcare safety. Paper presented at the Annual National Clinical Assessment Service Conference, March 2009, DfES.

Fawcett, J. (2013) Thoughts about multidisciplinary, interdisciplinary, and transdisciplinary research. *Nursing Science Quarterly*, 26(4), 376–79.

Harris, T. (1995) *I'm OK, You're OK*, 4th edition. Arrow Books.

Jelphs, K., Dickinson, H. and Miller, R. (2016) *Working in Teams*, 2nd edition. Policy Press.

Kilmann, R.H. and Thomas, K.W. (1977) Developing a forced-choice measure of conflict-handling behaviour: the MODE instrument. *Education and Psychological Measurement*, 37(2), 309–25.

Koprowska, J. (2010) *Communication and Interpersonal Skills in Social Work*, 3rd edition, Transforming Social Work Practice series. Learning Matters.

Laming, W. (2009) *The Protection of Children in England: a progress report*. The Stationery Office.

Morris, G., Prankard, S. and Lefroy, L. (2013) Animating experience: bringing student learning to life through animation and service user and carer experience. *Journal of Practice Teaching and Learning*, 12(1), 17–28.

Nursing and Midwifery Council (2018). *Future Nurse: standards of proficiency for registered nurses*, NMC. Available at: www.nmc.org.uk/globalassets/sitedocuments/education-standards/future-nurse-proficiencies.pdf (accessed 30 September 2019).

Tuckman, B.W. (1965) Developmental sequences in small groups. *Psychological Bulletin*, 63(6), 384–399.

Tuckman, B.W. and Jensen, M.A.C. (1977) Stages of small group development revisited. *Group and Organizational Studies*, 2(4), 419–27.

Weinstein, J. (2008) Working in partnership and collaboratively with other professionals. In Okitikpi, T. and Aymer, C. (eds) *The Art of Social Work Practice*. Russell House.

West, M.A., Borrill, C. and Unsworth, K. (1998) Team effectiveness in organizations. In Cooper, C.L. and Robinson, I.T. (eds) *International Review of Industrial and Organizational Psychology*, vol. 13. Wiley.

West, M.A. and Lyubovnikova, J. (2013) Illusions of team working in healthcare. *Journal of Health Organisation and Management*, 27(1), 134–42.

Chapter 11
Skills for presentations and public speaking

Paul Jeorrett

LEARNING OUTCOMES

When you have completed this chapter you should be able to:

11.1 Prepare, plan and practise your presentations

11.2 Deliver your presentations effectively and confidently.

11.1 Introduction

Presentations and public speaking are important in nearly all professional careers in the twenty-first century. Presentation skills are critical in communicating information, presenting and promoting you and your ideas and in sharing knowledge to groups of all sizes and in many contexts, at school, university, conferences and at career interview and recruitment processes. However, a YouGov poll showed that glossophobia, the fear of public speaking, was the third greatest fear for people in the UK (YouGov, 2014). In this chapter you will learn about some of the keys to preparing, planning and delivering an effective presentation which might help to overcome some of your fears. Having increased your confidence there is then no substitute for practice.

11.2 The 3 Ps: preparation, planning, practice

The 3Ps are general principles that you need to use in the lead up to delivering your presentation. They are applicable in all situations where you will be presenting something to an audience, either as an individual or as part of a group.

 IMPROVING RESILIENCE, LIFELONG LEARNING AND EMPLOYABILITY

By following these guidelines you will develop your study skills and improve your confidence in presenting information for employers, developing the lifelong learning skills to give a good presentation and be more resilient as you will be well prepared for most circumstances.

11.2.1 Preparation

There are several aspects that you need to consider when preparing a presentation, and you will soon discover that it takes many study skills to do so.

Who are you speaking to?

The first thing you need to consider is who your audience is. This is crucial in deciding how to focus your presentation. For example, you may prepare a presentation about caring for stroke patients for your tutor and fellow students as part of an assessment. However, your approach would be completely different if you were to do a similar presentation to a group of unknown health professionals as part of a seminar or conference.

Try to get a general idea of who will be in your audience beforehand. For example, you need to find out what your audience might already know and decide how best to deliver the information you want to give them. Also bear in mind equality and diversity issues such as gender, disability and cultural differences.

ACTIVITY 11.1
Think about a group you might have to do a presentation for. Consider the possible profile of your audience, taking into consideration issues relating to equality and diversity. How do you make your presentation as inclusive as possible?

What are you talking about?

What are the learning outcomes and what do you want your audience to do or remember as a result of your presentation? Have you been given a clear brief beforehand? If so, you need to ensure you are working closely to this. This will give you the key focus for your presentation and help you identify what might need to be included. For example, you have been asked to talk to school children about healthy lifestyles. To do this, you could design a few learning outcomes to be achieved by the end of the presentation. These might include:

Learning outcome 1 – What is a healthy lifestyle?
Learning outcome 2 – How can children make their lives more healthy?
Learning outcome 3 – How can adults help children to develop healthy lifestyles?

At the end of the presentation your audience should know the answers to these questions.

Gathering relevant data

Having decided who you are speaking to and what your key learning outcomes will be, you should gather all the relevant data you will need to ensure you know your subject thoroughly. Preparation for any presentation or speech should be the same as for any piece of research such as an essay, assignment or dissertation. Give yourself time using the study skills in this book to do a thorough literature review, exploiting the range of information sources such as books, journals, quality internet sources and reports.

(See *Chapter 3* for how to explore the literature.) In the era of 'fake news' it is important that your check your sources are reliable. Try using the CRAAP (Currency Relevance Authority Accuracy and Purpose) test on the sources you wish to use. It is also important to remember that in health and social sciences it is essential that you are able to present an evidence-based approach in many contexts. It is also important to ensure that you are able to use images, sound files and video in your presentation; a useful place to start is Creative Commons, where you can use files with appropriate attribution. For more information on how to use the CRAAP test, go to this library website: https://guides. library.illinoisstate.edu/evaluating/craap.

In relation to our above sample presentation, how would you apply the CRAAP test?
- Is the information you have on healthy eating **Current**?
- Is the information you are presenting **Relevant** to your audience?
- Is the information you are presenting from a good **Authority** or expert?
- Is the information you have **Accurate**?
- Does the information you have fit the **Purpose** of your presentation?

It is very easy to go off-track with your assignments and presentations so this tool might be a helpful way of remembering how to stay focused. Please also see *Chapter 3* on note-taking.

Prepare an outline and KISS

When you feel comfortable with who you are speaking to and what you are going to say, you should prepare a basic outline for your presentation. It is often helpful to think of your presentation as telling a story; think about how you might structure what you say to keep your audience interested. A good way to consider this is to watch TED Talks (www.ted.com/talks), where often complex information is transmitted in this style within a tight time constraint. Remember that most people can only concentrate for a maximum of 20 minutes. People respond better to presentations if they are both interested in the topic and involved in the presentation itself, so remember KISS – Keep It Simple and Straightforward. Don't try to explain huge amounts of theory in 10 minutes, or read out large blocks of text – you'll get lost and confused and your audience will get bored and frustrated. If you can, try to encourage audience participation, either through questions or activities depending on the circumstances, as this will help keep them engaged.

Using presentation software such as Microsoft PowerPoint, Google Slides or Prezi can be helpful at this stage, even if you are not going to use it for the presentation itself, as it works on the principle of a series of slides. This allows you to break down what you are going to say into manageable blocks of information which can be moved around and reworked as you develop the presentation. You may have your own system for approaching this depending on your personal preferences, such as a series of cardboard record cards or using a mind map (see *Chapter 3* on note-taking for how to create a mind map), so use whatever works best for you.

ACTIVITY 11.2

How would you go about gathering the information for a presentation? You might like to think about a subject you are about to research. Use the information in *Chapter 4* of this book to help you do a thorough literature review and then prepare an outline as if you were going to do a presentation. Try using the CRAAP test to check your sources. You might like to try this exercise working as a group and decide how you would divide the process up.

Presentations are a two-way process

The best presentations are a learning opportunity for both the audience and the presenter(s). If you are developing your own ideas it is invaluable to enter into a dialogue with the participants. Very often this will be through questions from the audience; it is your choice whether to field questions during your session or to take them at the end. Whatever you decide, make sure you inform the audience at the beginning.

During the preparation stage you should think about the questions your audience may have about the content of the presentation – and try to answer these during your presentation. Don't worry if you don't think of everything, as it is very hard to predict what questions may come up. However, you should be able to prepare for the majority of them; this approach will also help you when preparing for a job interview.

Where will the presentation take place and what equipment will be available?

You need to think about where the presentation will take place, as this will help you decide what equipment you might or might not use. If it is a university lecture theatre or classroom you will probably have full access to computers, projectors, screens, flip charts, etc. If you are presenting to a community group in a rural village hall you may only have your own voice to rely on, unless you can provide your own equipment. Don't feel pressured into using visual aids and equipment you are unfamiliar with; do what works for you!

It is probably best to imagine the worst-case scenario and work from that point. The worst thing that can happen is if there is a power cut, so if you can prepare for your presentation with this in mind you will be ready for anything! Always have notes or handouts for you and your audience; then at least you have a guide to what you are going to say and something for the audience to follow or to take away.

It is also a good idea to have a back-up plan if you want to use an online resource such as an online video demonstration as part of your presentation. Make sure you have an offline version available in case there is poor internet connectivity, or a set of slides showing the same steps as in the demonstration.

ACTIVITY 11.3

Think about a venue that you might have to give a presentation in. See if you can arrange with your tutor to use a suitable room to make this a practical exercise. What equipment will you use? Does it influence how you prepare for your presentation? Does the venue limit you or offer opportunities? What is the worst that could happen and how would you prepare for it?

11.2.2 Planning

All forms of communication should have a structure; otherwise, your main focus will be lost. Structure is important, and you will have already started to develop this in preparing an outline for your presentation. In any public speaking the essential advice is to have a beginning, a middle and an end. In short, say what you're going to say, say it; and then say what you have said. Each of these sections carries equal importance and has a clear role to play in the success of your presentation, as you will see.

 IMPROVING RESILIENCE, LIFELONG LEARNING AND EMPLOYABILITY

Presentation skills are important in helping you to demonstrate your knowledge to prospective employers. Once you have discovered how to demonstrate your learning in the classroom or at conferences you will be more confident when you start applying for that dream job.

The beginning

The beginning is crucial; in the first few moments the audience will decide whether they want to listen to you or not. So here are some tips to getting off to a good start:

- Do not hide but speak directly to the audience and make eye contact; if you are in a large room try and focus on the middle distance as this will make most people feel you are looking at them
- Start positively and engage the audience's attention, establishing a relationship with them
- Introduce yourself and smile as naturally as possible
- Introduce your topic and outline what you will be talking about
- Make each participant feel that you are speaking directly to them and that you want them to learn as a result of your presentation.

The middle

The middle section of your presentation contains the core of what you are going to say and will probably be the longest section. You will find it helpful to break this section down into subsections with an understandable sequence. As with your preparation, you may find presentation software helpful at this stage. Within a 20-minute presentation you will probably only be able to develop a maximum of five clear sections, although the ideal is probably about three. Most public speakers such as politicians, vicars, etc. will usually have three clear points to get over, as this is the most that an audience will probably remember. In our example above on the healthy eating presentation we had three learning outcomes that we wanted to achieve.

It is important to have a clear bridging link between each point; this can either be verbal, for instance, 'I would now like to move on to …' or a visual link using presentation software transitions or a simple hand gesture. This will enable you to lead the audience through what you have to say and keep them interested. Try not to labour each point as the audience will lose interest and you risk giving too much emphasis to one section over another. Remember people want to learn about you or from you and the presentation is your way of helping them do this. If you talk too much about one section they may forget what they have learnt about the other sections. It is important here to keep making the links for them and keep referring back to other sections in the presentation. This also helps you to develop and demonstrate your critical analysis skills, as outlined in *Chapter 5*.

The end

In the final section of your presentation you should try to provide a logical conclusion. These are some things you should try and do:

1. Give a brief summary of what you have said, emphasising the key points
2. Make sure you make it clear that you are finishing and ease into the end; don't just say, '… and that's it!' and walk away
3. It is better to begin your conclusion by saying '… and now I would like to finish by …'
4. Thank your audience
5. Don't forget to ask for any questions
6. Ensure that your audience goes away with something in their hands to remind them of what you have said, usually in the form of handouts
7. Give out evaluation sheets to make sure you get feedback to help you prepare for future presentations.

HELPFUL HINTS: WATCH YOUR OWN BEHAVIOUR

Breathe slowly and naturally – it is easy to forget to breathe normally in the heat of the moment.

Volume – you should look up as this will help you to speak up. If you keep your head down you will probably mumble and the audience won't hear you.

Don't shout; speak audibly and clearly. If you are asked to use a microphone, make sure it works and you hold or place it correctly and don't let it distract you.

Tone – the tone of your voice is important; if you speak in a monotone you will lose your audience's attention very quickly. If you smile you are more likely to sound enthusiastic and engaging; this doesn't come naturally to many of us and you will need to practise.

Pace – focus on the normal pace of your speech. Try not to speak too slowly or too fast so that you can breathe properly while presenting.

van Emden and Becker provide a 'Voice Checklist' that you may find useful (van Emden and Becker, 2016, p. 6):

- Is my voice loud, perhaps too loud?
- Is my voice soft, perhaps too soft?
- Do I speak too quickly?
- Do I speak too slowly?
- Is my voice monotonous?
- Do I articulate clearly or do I mutter?
- Will my accent cause my audience any particular difficulty?
- Do I run out of breath and gasp for air as I speak?

11.2.3 Practice

It is very important that you make time for the third P, practice. Having done the hard work of preparing and planning your presentation, it is absolutely essential that you rehearse and practise your performance thoroughly.

 IMPROVING RESILIENCE, LIFELONG LEARNING AND EMPLOYABILITY

Practice will help you to build your resilience to pre-presentation anxiety and to deal with unexpected events such as glitches in technology during your presentation.

How you practise is entirely down to personal preference, but here are a few suggestions:

- Record yourself reading through the presentation, concentrating on the volume and tone of your voice. This is tricky as it is always difficult listening to your own voice played back; however, this is what your audience will be listening to.
- Practise the timing of your presentation – are you trying to squeeze too much in? Do you move smoothly between each point? It is not good if you go over time and end up rushing through the last and probably most important bit of the presentation.
- Practise with any equipment you might be using, in front of willing volunteers. If you can do this in the venue you will be using, so much the better. Some students help each other to practise in the room they will be giving the presentation in. This helps them to gain confidence and obtain feedback.
- If you are using notes make sure that they are not intrusive and that they work for you.
- Learn the introduction to your presentation by heart; this will give you confidence in giving a good first impression.

It is important that you get feedback on your presentation, so ask your volunteers to evaluate you. If you have had feedback from presentations you have done previously, you can use this to fine-tune your performance. The following are some points you should consider when asking others to evaluate your performance or when evaluating your own performance:

- Were my points clear, interesting and in a logical structure?
- Are the pace and volume of the presentation right?
- Did I make a good first impression and was my body language appropriate?
- Did I connect with my audience using direct eye contact, interaction, etc.?
- Were the visual aids I used clear and not intrusive, and did I manage the equipment effectively?
- Was my conclusion handled well?

Stella Cottrell provides a very helpful self-evaluation sheet on 'How effective am I at talks/presentations?', which you might want to use when practising or as a basis for evaluation forms at the end of your presentation (Cottrell, 2019, p. 195).

Use your practice and evaluation to rework your presentation and ensure that all your notes and equipment work for you and you feel comfortable with them. You may still feel nervous, but you will certainly be more confident if you give yourself plenty of time to work through the three Ps.

ACTIVITY 11.4

As part of Graham's course assessment he has been asked to do a 20-minute presentation to the course group based on a topic that has been the main focus for the term. He is expected to use media to enhance his presentation where appropriate. Graham has never had to stand up and speak to a group before, or use media such as Microsoft PowerPoint, although he has had some experience of amateur dramatics. He is fine with researching and writing an assignment, but the thought of public speaking terrifies him.

How would you help Graham prepare for his presentation?

11.3 Delivering the presentation

So now the day of your presentation has arrived. Here are some guides to harnessing your performing edge, making a good impression, considering your vocal performance, controlling body language and using media and equipment. If you have practised as suggested above you will also probably now be aware of how good an impression you can make.

11.3.1 Harnessing your performing edge

It is quite normal to feel nervous when you are about to do something important and potentially challenging. If you do not feel a certain amount of anxiety before your presentation, whatever the situation, then you may not be as prepared as you thought. If you have followed the three Ps and given yourself plenty of preparation and practice time then you will go into the performance feeling more confident. However, here are a few tips:

- Use relaxation techniques if they help you, such as breathing exercises, t'ai chi, yoga, meditation or just sitting quietly.
- It is probably not a good idea to go on a wild night out the evening prior to your performance! Drinking too much alcohol just before you go on is definitely not a good idea. This can be challenging if you have been asked to speak following a conference dinner, but try and be restrained.
- The main tool you will be using during this exercise will be your voice, so try some warm-ups. van Emden and Becker (2016) offer some helpful vocal exercises in their book.
- Dress smartly but make sure that you are comfortable, because tight and restrictive clothes and shoes won't help you to relax.

11.3.2 Making a good first impression

Now you are confident and as relaxed as possible, it is time to walk on. It is important that you present yourself well; this doesn't mean you have to wear a suit, but it is helpful if you dress appropriately for the situation. Walk on confidently and smile if you can, make eye contact and you will form a rapport with your audience more quickly. The presentation begins from the moment you stand up.

 IMPROVING RESILIENCE, LIFELONG LEARNING AND EMPLOYABILITY

Presenting yourself well and making a good first impression will also be important when you are being interviewed for a job.

It is important to stand during your presentation. This will help you feel more confident, keep you alert and will allow you to project your voice more effectively. Remember, you should not try to hide; you are the main focus for the length of your presentation and anything else will be a distraction.

Before you begin, check that everyone can see and that they can all hear you. Try not to block any screens or flip charts that you are using and avoid extravagant body language before you begin.

As noted above, it is helpful if you can memorise the introduction to your presentation; this will get you off to a good start and help your confidence levels.

11.3.3 Your voice

Hopefully you will have learned to use your voice appropriately while practising your presentation; however, it is all too easy to forget this in the first anxious moments of standing up to begin. So remind yourself before your performance: if you speak too slowly, the audience will lose interest; too fast and what you say will not be understood and you will miss your key points.

- Avoid using jokes; they rarely work! If you need to use humour do it appropriately and don't force it; in this way it can be useful in keeping your audience's attention.
- Avoid slang, jargon and colloquialisms. Assume that you need to explain any technical language unless you are sure that your audience will all understand.
- Many people worry about 'drying up'. If this happens you should pause and take a few moments to find your place and regroup. You can also have some water with you to give you that space to collect your thoughts and to avoid literally drying up.

11.3.4 Body language

We all use body language in our everyday communication, but it is important to control your non-verbal communication while doing your presentation without making yourself feeling too restricted. Here are a few useful tips:

- Be aware of your gestures and don't fidget; waving your arms wildly or pointing at the projector screen can be very distracting.
- It is fine to move around, but don't pace up and down as this can often show you are anxious.

- You can use a prop such as a pen or a handout – it might keep your hands occupied. However, if you are nervous any papers you are holding will shake, or you might be tempted to hide behind them and you may start to fidget with your pen. So it might be better if you can go hands-free.
- Don't keep your hands in your pockets or slouch, as this looks unprofessional.

ACTIVITY 11.5

Think of a topic as a group and give yourself 1 minute each to do a presentation on a topic you are interested in. Prepare and plan a brief outline and structure and then do the presentation in front of the group. Get them to give you positive critical feedback on how you performed, paying particular attention to your voice, body language and first impressions. How did you feel? Did you use any techniques to harness your performing edge?

11.3.5 Using presentation software and other media and equipment to enhance your presentation

The use of presentation software, such as Microsoft PowerPoint™, Google Slides or Prezi for all types of presentation is almost ubiquitous. This applies a lot of pressure to use the software for any presentation that you may be asked to do. Although it is helpful to be able to use presentation software, it doesn't mean that you always have to, or any other equipment, unless it actively enhances what you have to say and doesn't act as a diversion or distraction. Often, if it is a short presentation, it is more powerful if you can feel confident enough to speak directly to your audience using a few visual images but without too many visual aids, as it is more immediate.

However, if you do need to use presentation software make sure that you have all the equipment available to you. You will usually need a laptop, tablet or PC (with appropriate software or app loaded) linked to a projector with a screen to project on. You may also require speakers linked to the PC, tablet or laptop if you are going to use sound clips or musical clips. You may also need an internet link if you wish to demonstrate a live website, although be warned, live online demonstrations don't always go to plan and add an unwelcome risk to your presentation if you are already feeling nervous.

There is not enough space here to go into the detail of getting started with presentation software, although if you already use word-processing software you will find it quite easy to use. The main difference is that presentation software works on the principle of a series of slides into which you can insert text, images, movie clips, etc. and you can animate the slides and transitions between them. It is particularly useful for:

- presenting images, graphs, diagrams and video clips, but only if they add value to what you are saying and, if well-timed, can keep your audience's attention
- helping to organise, structure and pace your presentation effectively a slide at a time in bite-sized chunks that the audience can take in

- providing a useful prompt for what you intend to say; if you feel confident enough you might be able to dispense with copious notes and be prompted by each slide
- printing notes with each slide for your own reference and handouts for the audience with each slide and space for notes.

HELPFUL HINTS: POLISHING YOUR PRESENTATION

If you decide to use presentation software, here are some useful tips to bear in mind:
- Use the 6, 7, 8 rule – no more than 6 lines to a slide, letters no less than 7 mm high (about 28–32 point), no more than 8–10 slides for a 10-minute presentation.
- Check your spelling on all slides.
- Be consistent, using the same font and background throughout if possible. Remember, using coloured text can be visually disastrous and black on white is too harsh for many people to read. Try to use clear black text, preferably Arial or a sans serif font, on a pastel-coloured background.
- Don't be too creative with pictures, sounds and animations. Many people who discover presentation software for the first time use all the gadgets available; always use them sparingly and only if they emphasise a point, otherwise they are very distracting. Be aware that some people can be distracted or can suffer motion sickness with animated software such as Prezi.
- Remember to pause between each slide or screen as you reveal each line of text or image. If you are rushing to get through the slides you have too many and you need to reduce the number.
- Don't put more than one idea on each slide or screen, or try to squeeze too much in; you can always use additional slides if necessary.
- Take a look at some examples of other people's presentations on websites such as www.slideshare.net.

Presentation software is not the only thing you can use to enhance your presentation. You can use whiteboards (interactive or otherwise), blackboards and flipcharts to write comments from the audience and introduce some activity to keep everyone participating. In the following activity, spend some time thinking about what equipment you will need and how you will obtain it.

ACTIVITY 11.6

Find out what equipment might be available to you. Try and practise using presentation software and a range of other equipment and interactive techniques so that you become familiar with them, if you haven't already done so. If possible, incorporate them into some of the exercises mentioned above.

11.4 **Conclusion**

As a student in health and social care you will be asked to present your ideas sooner or later. This is because you will need to be able to do this as a professional and in some situations on behalf of the people you are caring for. Practice is one of the most important things you can do to help you develop presentation skills and using the activities within this chapter will guide you on what and how you should practise.

SUMMARY

Four key points to take away from *Chapter 11*:

- ☑ **Preparation** is important for finding out where and to whom you will be presenting.
- ☑ **Preparation** will help you to keep it simple and straightforward (KISS).
- ☑ **Planning** helps you to find tools that will help you give a great presentation.
- ☑ **Practice** helps you to make time to develop your skills and confidence.

Quiz

1. What are the 3 Ps you should remember when preparing a presentation?
2. How can you improve your presentation skills using lifelong learning?
3. How can you improve your employability skills using presentations?
4. How can you become more resilient when giving presentations?

REFERENCES

Cottrell, S. (2019) *The Study Skills Handbook*, 5th edition. Palgrave Macmillan.

van Emden, J. and Becker, L. (2016) *Presentation Skills for Students*, 3rd edition. Palgrave Macmillan.

YouGov (2014) YouGov reveals what scares Britain (heights) – and what doesn't (Clowns). Available at https://yougov.co.uk/topics/politics/articles-reports/2014/03/20/afraid-heights-not-alone (accessed 9 September 2019).

Chapter 12
Skills for employability in health and social care

Marjorie Ghisoni

LEARNING OUTCOMES

When you have completed this chapter you should be able to:

12.1 Demonstrate key skills that are useful for employability

12.2 Discuss how employability skills are influenced by lifelong learning

12.3 Identify how resilience skills can support employability

12.4 Make a start on producing your own portfolio of professional development.

12.1 Introduction

In this chapter we will explore how you can develop your employability skills as you study so that when you complete your course, you will be able to find work quickly and confidently in the health and social care services. When you decide to choose a course of study you may be thinking about what area of health and social care services you would like to work in. Some people may not know at this stage and are happy to wait until the end of the course before deciding on their employment options, but others may know already before starting the course where they want to work. This chapter will help you to identify the skills you will need to develop so that you can be confident in finding employment in your chosen career.

Wherever you decide to work, you will need to be equipped with some of the skills already discussed in this book and in particular where other chapters discuss employability. For example, in *Chapter 9* you are required to think critically about your practice or experiences and to reflect upon them so that you can learn from them. This might also affect your employability skills because it requires you to focus your attention on what skills you will need. You may be required to work with many other people or just a few. You might also be required to work with different professional groups and organisations. This might appear daunting, but it is the nature of many health and social care services where most staff are required to work in a multidisciplinary or interprofessional way.

In *Chapter 10* you are asked to look at your teamworking skills in some depth so that you will be prepared, by developing your resilience and employability skills, to work in different environments with different people. This chapter will discuss in more detail how you can use your study skills in health and social care to improve your employability prospects. We will use your lifelong learning and resilience skills to help you to do this.

12.2 Developing employability skills using your lifelong learning skills

In *Chapter 9* we discussed how reflective practice can help you to develop your knowledge and skills for practice and how graduateness can be a way of improving your employability. Most students take a great deal of time preparing for their higher education and may have already discussed with other professionals where they would like to find employment in the health and social care sector. For many professionals education does not end once they have found employment, and when applying for interviews it is useful to consider your lifelong learning needs. The opportunities for lifelong learning offered in a particular post may help you to choose where you would like to work if you have already given it prior consideration, and prospective employers may be quite impressed if you have thought this far ahead. After all, if you are prepared to continually develop yourself then that might influence other staff who might then want to improve the service they deliver.

Health and social care is a fast-changing profession, with people working more and more in a multidisciplinary way. Often staff from different disciplines in healthcare might find themselves working with staff from completely different professions. In *Chapter 10* you will already have looked at the importance of teamworking, but if you can demonstrate that you are aware of such different ways of working, then it will increase your employability in the health and social care field.

ACTIVITY 12.1

Consider what skills you will need to demonstrate and improve your employability with prospective organisations. Make a list below to help you review your individual employability skills using the chapters of this book to help you, e.g. I am good at searching the literature to keep my knowledge and practice up to date.

My individual list of employability skills

Now that you have your list it can act as a reminder to you on how you want to develop your individual skills. If you struggle to find skills to add to your list, you might want to discuss with a friend or mentor who can help you to see where you have good skills in lifelong learning. Don't worry if you become aware of skills that also need developing, as you will be able to reflect upon these later and find ways to improve them. Having a variety of lifelong learning skills will help you to become more confident in your knowledge base and more confident in your ability to future-proof your employability skills.

HELPFUL HINT

Most courses provide students with personal tutors who you can talk to about anything that is affecting your studies, but when you go out into practice you should still use this resource to aid your development. Some students develop peer-support networks and it might be worth joining them to offer and find support outside of work or education. Try to find a social media group in your area of practice and if it is online you can also use it to develop your professional profile for future employers.

12.3 Key lifelong learning skills for employability

Even if you have never experienced the working environment there will be certain lifelong learning skills that you will be required to demonstrate at interview and in practice. However, these are skills that you are developing all of the time as you learn to live and work with other people in the family environment and in the education environment.

HELPFUL HINT

Think about the times when you are in lectures and the tutor asks you to discuss an idea with your peers in small groups. This is a good way to help you put your thoughts and new-found knowledge into words. Many students and professionals find this very difficult to do, but it can also be practised using social media. See below for more advice on how to do this.

ACTIVITY 12.2

Think about some of the areas of your life where you have had to work or live with other people. We have already identified the first two as being:
The family and the wider family – e.g. aunts and uncles and grandparents
The school environment – e.g. teachers, school friends, administrators and housekeeping staff

You might also want to think about:
When you are on holiday
When you use public transport
When you are part of community groups

Now in the box below, think about what lifelong learning skills you use in each of these groups:

Group	Skills
Family	e.g. communication and relationship development skills
Work	e.g. communication and teamworking skills
Students	
Friends	
Community/social groups	
Hobbies/interests	
Holiday	
Travelling	
Public services, e.g. hospital/local council	
Other	

You may have identified skills such as good manners, communication skills, etc. These are sometimes called invisible skills or soft skills that are just as important in the working environment as the knowledge and skills that you develop around health and social care. In our everyday lives, however, we are often not aware of how employability skills are actually affecting our interactions with other people. If when we are trying to find work we are too shy to talk to people, for example, we will find it much harder to find employment. People who work in education such as tutors and lecturers are therefore required to help students develop employability skills so that they are ready for work when they have completed their course or education. When your tutor asks you to ask questions in class or discuss your ideas in a seminar, they are helping you to develop your employability skills.

12.4 Employability skills and professional practice

Higher education courses often do not discuss professional practice as part of the course curriculum, but there is some expectation that students will automatically develop this as they learn. This is where reflective practice can help you to work on your professional practice skills and begin to develop your own professional values and boundaries that will help you to identify what employability skills you need for where you want to eventually work.

Professional relationships are different from the other relationships that you have in your life, and if you are not prepared for them, you can risk breaching your professional code of practice. As you move closer to the end of your course you will be expected to be able to think critically about your professional practice using your skills of reflection so that you can demonstrate your knowledge and skills to become a safe and effective health and social care professional. Prospective employers will be looking for how you have developed as a professional and what skills and knowledge you have used to do this. In *Chapter 13* we will look at this in more depth.

HELPFUL HINT

Students and professionals are encouraged to demonstrate good professional practice in public as well as in the workplace. This includes when you go out to parties as well as talking to people online. Developing a blog can help you to do this as it will make you consider whether you are being professional and whether you are demonstrating up-to-date knowledge and skills.

In *Chapter 9* we discussed the importance of developing reflective practice skills for employability, but for this chapter we will focus upon the skills of reflection as a way of helping people to achieve their goals, in relation to employment opportunities. A SWOT (Strengths, Weaknesses, Opportunities, Threats) analysis is a useful way of exploring our individual strengths and weaknesses and identifying what might prevent us (threats) from moving smoothly along our chosen career pathway. In order to be able to develop ourselves and our skills we will also need to identify what choices we have (opportunities) and who will help us to access them – this could be a practice supervisor or a personal tutor. Consider the following examples in the SWOT analysis in *Activity 12.3* and then add some more of your own. Remember that strengths and weaknesses are internal and personal to you, and opportunities and threats are external.

ACTIVITY 12.3

Complete the SWOT analysis below.

Strengths *What do you know about your own strengths?*	e.g. I am good at listening
Weaknesses *What do you know about your own weaknesses?*	e.g. My concentration is poor sometimes
Opportunities *What opportunities do you have to develop your skills?*	e.g. My university has a great library to work in
Threats *What threats might prevent you from developing your skills?*	e.g. I don't have much money to get the bus to the library

Identifying and using or making visible your lifelong learning skills is a good way of demonstrating your employability to prospective employers or when you go for an interview for a professional course such as nursing, social work or psychology. They will also help you to develop your resilience skills.

12.5 **Developing resilience skills to improve your employability**

When we are developing our employability skills we are at the same time developing our skills of resilience. In *Chapter 1* we have discussed resilience in much more detail, but it is also a feature of this book in every chapter because we believe that it is a core skill in the essential skill set for health and social care. However, when we talk about resilience and employability we must think about it in a slightly different way. In relation to preparing ourselves for the health and social care workplace, or indeed any workplace, our resilience skills can help us to reflect upon what we might need to demonstrate at interview or in application letters to prospective employers.

Taylor (2016, p. 1) defines employability as 'the process of equipping yourself to be able to apply for and fulfil the personal specifications of a job'.

Resilience helps us to prepare ourselves for our future employment by becoming more aware of our needs and being more self-compassionate about our abilities and strengths (Ghisoni, 2016). In *Chapter 1* we identified Resilience as being a way of taking care of ourselves using Rest, Relaxation, Replenishment, Reflection and Respiration (the 5Rs). These five things that we do each day can become a good habit to get into by becoming mindful of how we are addressing our own resilience skills each day. They could be remembered by calling them your five-a-day for resilience so that you do not forget to check in with yourself to see how you are doing. When you are attending interviews for courses or employment you will need to demonstrate how you take care of yourself as well as your lifelong learning skills for employability. In *Activity 12.4* you can reflect upon what skills you might need to help you to do this.

ACTIVITY 12.4

From what you have read so far, try to think of some resilience skills that you might need to be successful in your chosen career (we have added some suggestions at the end of this chapter).

Resilience skills that I might need:

e.g. to learn how to cook better so that I eat more healthily (replenishment)

In the above activity you may have identified some very personal skills that you need to develop so that you can be more resilient in your everyday life and so that you can give your best efforts in your assignments or new employment. If we cannot take care of ourselves it will be very difficult for us to take care of the more vulnerable people that we might eventually be working with (Ghisoni, 2016). When we complete professional courses this is something that is not addressed very well and can lead to attrition or students leaving the course before they have completed it. Monitoring attrition rates is very important to educational establishments as well as other organisations, because a high attrition rate means a high staff or student turnover, which costs money and time to redress. Many organisations now want to know that you have developed resilience when you complete your course and many universities are focusing on student support services to help people to take more care of themselves.

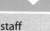

HELPFUL HINT

Before you apply for a course or a job check out how supportive the organisation is of its staff or students. Most universities or large organisations will have information on their student/staff support services available. As an example, see the website below for a range of support services available in most universities.

AMOSSHE Resilience Toolkit, https://resiliencetoolkit.org.uk

12.5.1 Developing resilience for employability as graduateness

Resilience in relation to education and employability is often referred to as 'graduateness'. This term implies that when you have completed a period of study, you not only have a qualification but you are also prepared as graduates for the field of work. Working in health and social care can be very stressful at times, but it is also a very rewarding occupation when you have dealt with a difficult situation to the best of your ability. Health professionals are expected to be critical thinkers and confident doers, who can think for themselves in any situation.

Consequently, Ramsey and Monk (2017) suggest that graduateness, measured through assessment, is becoming a more prominent requirement of many professional courses in health and social care. Students are often required to complete a portfolio of evidence so that prospective employers can see that you have developed your learning through reflection and continuous professional development.

12.5.2 What does a portfolio of evidence look like?

For many people a portfolio of evidence is simply a curriculum vitae (CV) that is regularly kept up to date. It is important that it is kept up to date so that when the opportunity to apply for that dream job arrives you are able to complete the application form quickly and confidently. For our own professional development we are often required by our professional bodies to produce more than a CV so that we can demonstrate learning has actually taken place. More and more prospective employers are wanting to see this type of portfolio rather than a list of previous employment or conferences attended. Many employers within the health and social care field are wanting to see what we can do for the organisation so that they can improve the service that they currently offer. This is very important in the rapidly changing world of health and social care (Taylor, 2016).

A portfolio of evidence is your way of showing that you can do the job based on the experience that you already have. In Nursing this is also a professional requirement so that you can remain in the professional register. Developing a portfolio of evidence is therefore a really important employability skill, but we also use our lifelong learning and resilience skills to put it together. The Open University offers free advice and short courses on many topics through their Open Learn site (www.open.edu/openlearn) which you can use to develop your skills further. They suggest that a portfolio of evidence should include:

A personal statement of you as a person: what you like to do and what you like to learn
  about. Try to keep this positive and start selling yourself as enthusiastic and willing to
  learn straight away.
Certificates and awards: these are your evidence of what you have achieved so far,
  so keep them safe.
A record of any experiences you have had where you can demonstrate your employability
  skills, such as volunteering in similar places of work or organisations.
Any reports or presentations you have produced demonstrating your employability skills.
Photographs of you or your achievements which is a good way to demonstrate your
  resilience skills, e.g. completing a sponsored walk or run for a local charity.
Published articles about you or that you have written: this demonstrates your lifelong
  learning and resilience skills.
References or statements of good character from your tutors or employers.

HELPFUL HINT ✔

Look at your own college or university guidelines on professional portfolio development and make a head start on producing your individual portfolio to demonstrate your employability skills to your next employer.

12.6 Developing transferable skills for employability

As suggested above, transferable skills are those that you can develop and take with you wherever you work and may be considered more important than knowledge development. In contrast, knowledge development often needs updating because new policy and research are incorporated into your body of evidence-based practice. Transferable skills, however, are something you develop on the job. You are continually practising them and they are probably the most important part of graduateness once you have completed your education. From the exercise above, make a note of what transferable skills you are good at and what skills are missing from your list. You can cross-reference this with the list of resilience skills for employability at the end of this chapter.

HELPFUL HINT: GO PEOPLE-WATCHING!

People-watching can be an art that we develop without even thinking about it, but it is also something we can learn a great deal from. When thinking about developing your skills for employability, spend some time observing in everyday practice how people you admire demonstrate their employability skills. You could also use this exercise as a reflection on your own employability skills.

Watch how they communicate with other people.

Do they look like they enjoy what they are doing?

Watch how they use their own body language to communicate with other people.

Do they talk about their employability skills without being overbearing?

Are they able to relate to the other person using compassion and empathy to demonstrate their understanding?

When we go about our daily lives we take little notice of what is going on around us. This is because we need to stay focused on getting from A to B. If we took notice of everything then we would probably never get anywhere. However, in order to identify and tell other people about our employability skills we need to be able to check in from time to time. You can do this as part of your reflective writing skills that were discussed in more detail in *Chapter 9*. In this chapter we look at some of the activities that have helped you to do this and explore some of the instinctual things that you do every day. As discussed above, these skills are often invisible to yourself as well as others unless you think about them in more detail using your skills of reflection and resilience to direct and support your lifelong learning.

ACTIVITY 12.5: DEVELOPING TRANSFERABLE RESILIENCE SKILLS FOR EMPLOYABILITY

Consider the following scenario:

John is a social worker with many years' experience in children's services, but now he wants to work in mental health services where he will be working with adults up to old age. He is wondering what skills he has that can be transferred to a new field of practice and needs to think about how he can demonstrate that he has something to offer, if and when he gets to interview.

List below five skills you think John might be able to transfer to his new job when he gets it.

1.

2.

3.

4.

5.

The knowledge that we develop from these invisible skills is known as 'tacit knowledge', which usually means that we know we have it but we don't know where it has come from. Yet, this is probably one of the most important parts of our employability skills because it is often based in experience. Many students are asked to keep a reflective journal or blog of their learning from experience to help them to identify quickly how they have learnt a new skill and what information supported it. This is a good practice to get into and it is a good way of organising your thoughts around something that you may want to revisit later in your career.

After 20 years of studying in my own professional life I realised upon reflection that I had no way of keeping all of this learning in one place. Collecting certificates is nice, but it does not really demonstrate what you have learnt to employers or others. Many prospective employers will search online for any person who has applied for jobs to check out their professionalism and experience and knowledge. Using social media can help us to do this, but it is important to be aware of Netiquette around posting anything online. Some of the main things you should consider when demonstrating your transferable skills for employability are listed in *Table 12.1*.

Table 12.1 *Ten dos and don'ts of developing employability skills using social media*

Dos	Don'ts
Do be polite and do not rant on about your beliefs and values	Don't shout at someone by writing in CAPITALS
Do leave comments where you can, to enter into a discussion and give feedback	Don't joke as it often backfires and causes offence
Do network on social media to help you develop your knowledge and career prospects	Don't be offensive, call people names or dismiss their comments as silly or stupid
Do greet and thank people as you would if it were a face-to-face meeting	Don't forget to check your spelling before sending a comment
Do post pictures and links, but always make sure they are respectful and confidential to others	Don't spend too much of your time on social media when you should be studying/working

Some professional organisations have produced guidelines on the professional use of social media, as it can be the leading cause of disciplinary action in some professions. For an example, see the Nursing and Midwifery Council Guidelines at www.nmc.org.uk/globalassets/sitedocuments/nmc-publications/social-media-guidance.pdf

For more information on how to develop your employability skills online, the following platforms are used by professionals to network with others in the same field of practice. Some universities and colleges are also using these to support students when they are off campus.

LinkedIn – www.linkedin.com
Twitter – https://twitter.com
ResearchGate –www.researchgate.com

12.7 **Conclusion**

In this chapter we have looked at how employability skills can help us to grow and develop in health and social care practice. While you are probably only focused upon your study skills right now, thinking about your further development can also help you to decide what skills to develop as you study. We have identified above that employability is becoming an increasingly important skill in the busy world of health and social care. Developing your skills in leadership and lifelong learning will help you to be more confident, not just about your learning but also for your future career in health and social care.

SUMMARY

Four key points to take away from *Chapter 12*:
- ☑ Good employability skills will help you feel more confident in getting that dream job.
- ☑ Becoming aware of your own employability skills helps you to become more resilient.
- ☑ Practising employability skills helps you to plan your career pathway.
- ☑ Developing a portfolio will help you prepare for applying for jobs.

Suggestions for resilience skills in employability

1. Confident in your knowledge.
2. Good communication skills.
3. Good problem-solving skills.
4. Good skills of reflection.
5. Good critical thinking skills.
6. Good teamworking skills.
7. Friendly and approachable.
8. Good literature-searching skills.
9. Knowledge of the process and application of research.
10. Quality improvement.

Quiz

1. What are employability skills?
   a. Skills that help you to get a job
   b. Skills that help you to study
   c. Skills that help you make good notes

2. What does a SWOT analysis mean?
   a. Strengths, Weaknesses, Organisations, Threats
   b. Support, Weaknesses, Opportunities, Threats
   c. Strengths, Weaknesses, Opportunities, Threats

3. Why do you need a portfolio of evidence?
   a. To demonstrate your graduateness
   b. To demonstrate your writing skills
   c. To demonstrate your reflective practice skills

4. How can social media help you to develop employability skills?
   a. By helping you to communicate with your peers
   b. By helping you to develop your computer skills
   c. By helping you to practise your knowledge

REFERENCES

Ghisoni, M. (2016) The components of compassion. In Hewison, A. and Sawbridge, Y. (eds) *Compassion in Nursing: theory, evidence and practice*. Oxford University Press.

Ramsey, M. and Monk, E. (2017) The professional graduate. In Normand, C. and Anderson, L. (eds) *Graduate Attributes in Higher Education*. Routledge.

Taylor, L. (2016) *How to Develop Your Healthcare Career: a guide to employability and professional development*. Wiley Blackwell.

Chapter 13
Skills for the developing professional

Marjorie Ghisoni

LEARNING OUTCOMES

When you have completed this chapter you should be able to:

13.1 Demonstrate professional skills for lifelong learning

13.2 Discuss how professional skills are important for employability

13.3 Identify resilience skills for professional development.

13.1 Introduction

… it should be recognised that health and social care professionals will have two sets of values; their professional values and their personal values, both of which can impact on the teams and organisation within which they are working.

(Jones and Bennett, 2018, p. 48)

In this chapter we will explore why it is important to develop your skills as a professional practitioner and how this can help you to find employment in the field of health and social care. As the above quote suggests, developing as a professional requires people to develop and understand the values of all the other professionals that they will be working with as well as their own. In addition, we bring to our professional practice personal values that we have held all of our lives and these may be based in cultural or personal beliefs. When we commence our studies in health and social care we are already bringing with us values and beliefs that we may need to challenge and explore as we develop our professional skills.

In order to develop your professional practice after you have completed your professional course, you will need to have resilience, lifelong learning and employability skills so that you can confidently apply your knowledge to your practice while coping in a very busy and sometimes very stressful professional world. We will explore further below how we can develop those skills, which as you will see are closely linked to other skills in this book such as critical thinking and teamworking.

13.2 **Developing resilience as a professional**

As Jones and Bennett (2018) suggest in the quote at the beginning of this chapter, as professionals we have personal, as well as professional, values to help us make decisions about our everyday practice. Some of those professional values are stated in codes of conduct or ethics by different professional bodies and we must pay close attention to them to remain registered as a professional practitioner. Therefore, it is important to familiarise yourself with them very quickly.

In a recent study on resilience in primary care staff (mainly doctors), it was found that workload management was an important factor in developing professional resilience. Robertson *et al.* (2016) found that professionals who had clear boundaries between their work and home life appeared to be more resilient, but they argue that more measurement is needed. Measuring professional resilience does not need to be long or time-consuming because this might only add to the stress that people are already under. Instead, a more compassionate approach to taking the time to ask your co-workers if they are okay or indeed to ask for help yourself can prevent people becoming fatigued and burnt out.

However, Robertson *et al.* (2016) suggest that professional resilience is multifaceted and can be developed in both our home and work lives. For example, learning how to manage stress and reflecting regularly upon our work will help us to identify early warning signs and the skills or resources to help us manage them. For more information on developing reflective writing skills see *Chapter 9*.

ACTIVITY 13.1: USING PROFESSIONAL CODES TO HELP BUILD RESILIENCE

What professional codes might you need to be aware of on your professional course? Remember, you might also need to be aware of other professionals that you will be working with. List the professional codes that you can find here:

1.

2.

3.

4.

Professional codes can be traced back to early medical history when practising doctors took the Hippocratic oath of *First Do No Harm*. Oxtoby (2016) suggests that this is a misquote of the original oath, but nevertheless it still holds as a moral compass for practising doctors today. This suggests that professional and personal values may be very closely interlinked and that both should focus upon developing caring relationships in practice. This applies to caring relationships with our colleagues as well as ourselves.

Therefore, resilience in professional development must be focused upon our ability to care for ourselves and others in such a way that we do not harm. This also links this area of our practice with our reflective practice that is discussed in *Chapter 9*. In order to develop self-awareness around our values, beliefs and coping skills as a professional, we will need to take some time to reflect.

ACTIVITY 13.2: RECOGNISING PERSONAL AND PROFESSIONAL VALUES

Consider the following scenario and what personal and professional values this person might need to reflect upon.

Sally worked in a busy multidisciplinary team as a junior nurse. She had not long qualified and was eager to put into practice all that she had learnt over the last three years of her nurse education. At the team meeting a referral came in for a lady who was struggling to look after her children after developing severe depression. There was a concern that the children were being neglected, as their school reported them arriving unwashed and poorly dressed. Sally was feeling anxious about the children and the harm they might come to and she was struggling to understand why the mother was not getting help for her children.

What values might Sally be expressing/thinking?
- Personal values of what family life should be like?
- Professional values of taking care of people who cannot do it for themselves?
- Professional values of sharing concerns with other members of the team?
- Personal values of what a good mother should look like?

Professional values are an important part of our working lives, but they also become part of our personal lives as we must always act as professional people as we develop our career working lives. It is therefore important to develop a good work–life balance so that we can be mindful of our values and beliefs at all times. It is, however, easy to overstep professional boundaries, and this can get us into trouble with our professional bodies.

13.2.1 Professional misconduct

Professional misconduct applies to anything that we do that could undermine the public's confidence in us as professionals. This might include our behaviour in or out of the work areas. Professional bodies such as the NMC (2018a) have produced a code of conduct to help us to be aware of our behaviour and to reflect all of the time on how we behave. *Chapter 9* helps us to develop skills of reflection, but we also need to think about our professional codes in many areas of our lives as a student and a practitioner. Some of the areas we may not consider at risk are often the areas that are most often breached, e.g.
- Driving at speed and risking lives
- Taking illegal drugs
- Getting drunk in public
- Failing to document something correctly
- Failing to report something to managers
- Becoming too friendly with patients or clients
- Abusing the trust of carers or patients
- Violence or aggression in the workplace or in public
- Misuse of social networking sites
- Developing inappropriate relationships.

There are probably many more than can be listed here, but it is worth taking some time to consider your professional boundaries and how they might impact on your personal and professional life (General Social Care Council, 2011).

13.2.2 The influence of student misconduct on professional development and resilience

Most universities and colleges have policies around student misconduct which could affect your ability to study and complete your course, so it is very important to become familiar with these polices so that you learn and practise safely at all times. If you are studying for a professional award you will also need to adhere to professional codes as outlined above. For students you might think it is not such an issue while you are in university or college, but it can affect your references for jobs at a later date. As lecturers in a professional field we are required to provide references of good character to our professional bodies so that they are sure that upon completion of a professional course you are fit and safe to practise. You will then be given a PIN number to show that you are registered as a professional practitioner. This registration also has to be renewed every few years – for example, the NMC requires nurses to revalidate every three years – and you will more often than not be required to demonstrate evidence of further learning, usually by some reflective accounts. Therefore, it is important that as a student you get into good habits now.

Often students get into trouble through not knowing what academic misconduct is and rarely because they are deliberately cheating or causing harm. However, the availability of internet search engines and social media and the risk of plagiarism can sometimes turn an enjoyable assignment into a nightmare. Please see *Chapter 7* for more information on how to reference your work correctly. We have also discussed the safe use of social media in the previous chapter.

Consider the following scenario which may be familiar to you in education, but remember this can happen to professionals too, especially when they are rushing to meet publication deadlines. In some countries staff are dependent on publications to keep their jobs, so it is a lifelong skill as well as a resilience and employability skill to remain professional at all times.

ACTIVITY 13.3: DEVELOPING RESILIENCE AROUND ACADEMIC MISCONDUCT

Sumar was aiming for a first-class degree because she wanted to continue her professional career and train to be a doctor. Sumar was usually quite organised, giving herself plenty of time to complete and check her assignments. However, she had been quite unwell and had not been able to stay as focused on her studies as she usually was. Sumar asked a friend if she could look at their work to check that she was doing it right. Sumar trusted this friend and knew they were quite good academically. The friend agreed and sent her a copy by email. Sumar followed her friend's outline, listing the main learning outcomes for the assignment and she borrowed some references as she would probably have found the same ones anyway. When the assignment was returned after marking it was a fail due to plagiarism. Sumar was very upset, but did not know what she had done wrong.

Sumar did not intend to cheat – in fact, that was the last thing on her mind – so she was devastated when she realised people thought this of her. How could you advise Sumar to prevent this happening again?

Here are some pieces of advice that you might have thought of:
- Don't look at other people's work because you could copy it by mistake

- Don't copy other people's work even if you intend to change the wording, as it could still be picked up by plagiarism software
- Talk to your personal tutor if you think you are not going to meet a deadline
- Don't copy and paste information even with a reference – it is still not your work
- Don't copy references, as this can give you a high plagiarism score.

HELPFUL HINT

If you are worried about plagiarism you need to learn more about it and practise checking your assignments often. Most universities and colleges allow you to do this before you submit the final draft. Try using free plagiarism software such as those mentioned below so that you can check your assignments as often as you want. They sometimes also offers free plagiarism advice.
VIPER – www.scanmyessay.com
Quetex – www.quetext.com

13.3 Developing employability skills in professional practice

In *Chapter 12* we briefly looked at developing professional practice as part of our employability skills. Here we will look at this in more depth and identify some ways that we can develop resilience in our professional practice.

Winbolt (2016) suggests that there are some ways in which we can all develop resilience and employability skills in our workplace to demonstrate professional practice. In demonstrating that we are aware of this, our prospective employers will also be aware that we recognise it. We may not always observe our own behaviour in as much detail as we are asking you to do in this book, but when we practise these skills in self-monitoring and self-compassion, we are becoming mindful of our values and attitudes in our personal and professional lives. Once we are more confident of our employability skills and that we are able to present ourselves as 'graduates', we will also demonstrate that we are confident in our knowledge and skills in our professional practice.

ACTIVITY 13.4

Consider the following ways of building resilience at work outlined by Winbolt (2016) and reflect upon how many you already use in your everyday life.

Nine ways to build resilience at work (Winbolt, 2016):
1. *Cherish social support and interaction.* Good relationships with family and friends and others are vital. Being active in the wider community also helps.
2. *Treat problems as a learning process.* Develop the habit of using challenges as opportunities to acquire or master skills and build achievement.
3. *Avoid making a drama out of a crisis.* Stress and change are part of life. How we interpret and respond to events has a big impact on how stressful we find them.
4. *Celebrate your successes.* Take time at the end of each day to review what went well and congratulate yourself. This trains the mind to look for success rather than dwelling on negativity and 'failure'.
5. *Develop realistic life goals for guidance and a sense of purpose.* Do something each day to move towards them. Again, small is beautiful; one small step amid the chaos of a busy day will help.

6. *Take positive action.* Doing something in the face of adversity brings a sense of control, even if it doesn't remove the difficulty.
7. *Nurture a positive view of yourself.* Developing confidence in your ability to solve problems and trusting your instincts helps to build resiliency.
8. *Keep a realistic perspective.* Place challenging or painful events in the broader context of life-long personal development.
9. *Practise optimism.* Nothing is either wholly good or bad. If we allow our thinking to dictate how we view something, it will take over. Make your thinking work for your benefit, rather than letting it stymie you with doubt or by seeing only the bad side.

You may find it difficult to relate to the above ways of building employability skills using resilience at work if you are not used to reflective practice or you may not have been in the working environment yet, so we have included an example below.

EXAMPLE 13.1: DEVELOPING RESILIENCE IN PROFESSIONAL PRACTICE

Bob is a social worker with a busy caseload of adults from the ages of 18 to 65. Bob enjoys his job because it is very varied, but some days he feels very overwhelmed with his work. He has tried discussing it with his manager, but they are very busy too. When Bob gets home from work he is too tired to take care of himself properly. He often goes straight to bed, but is still having trouble sleeping and wakes in the morning and goes to work exhausted.

We can apply the nine ways of resilience to Bob's situation as outlined below.
1. Bob has lost a lot of his relationships because he no longer goes out.
2. Bob see his problems as hopeless, not as opportunities to develop new skills.
3. Bob finds his professional role very hard and stressful.
4. Bob does not see or reflect upon the success he has made in his job.
5. Bob does not make realistic plans because he is often overwhelmed with his workload.
6. Bob does not see how he can change things because he is often too exhausted.
7. Bob is losing confidence in his ability to do his job well.
8. Bob cannot see how to change things and is not reflecting upon his practice.
9. Bob is not very optimistic because he is feeling so hopeless.

Demonstrating resilience for employability is important, because prospective employers will see you as a professional and reliable practitioner and, perhaps, a potential leader. When you demonstrate resilience in the workplace, whether as a student on a practice placement or as an employee in practice, you are also modelling these skills for others and thus helping them to develop their own resilience and improve their own practice. You can also use the 5Rs for resilience in *Chapter 1* to help you to remember to look after yourself.

HELPFUL HINT

Keeping a reflective journal, diary or blog will help us to record our thoughts, reflections and observations so that we do not forget them and can use them for revalidation purposes when we need to. Many education organisations encourage students to get into this habit early either through keeping a reflective portfolio of their studies or an online blog, which in some universities and colleges contribute to their assessment marks. See *Chapter 12* for more information on keeping a portfolio.

13.3.1 How does evidence-based practice support professional development?

All health and social care practitioners are expected to be able to demonstrate their knowledge base for their practice, otherwise they could be not practising safely. This is known as evidence-based practice (EBP) and is a requirement of most professional fields in order to maintain a valid professional qualification and/or registration. Heaslip and Lindsay (2019) suggest that EBP 'involves using the best evidence you have about the most effective care of individuals, using it with the person's best interests in mind, to the best of your ability and in such a way that it is clear to others that you are doing it'. EBP also contributes to our continuous professional development, which will be discussed later in this chapter.

When people are hurt or distressed, however, they do not think about how much knowledge you have – they just want you to make them feel better. This can pose a dilemma for you as a health and social care practitioner, because most of us come into these professions because we want to help people. Again, our professional codes of conduct and standards of proficiency can help us here and can be used to support your academic work. For example, according to *Future Nurse: standards of proficiency for registered nurses* (NMC, 2018b), a qualified nurse must:

- demonstrate an understanding of research methods, ethics and governance in order to critically analyse, safely use, share and apply research findings to promote and inform best nursing practice
- safely demonstrate evidence-based practice in all skills and procedures.

In the same way, social workers must 'recognise the value of research and analysis and be able to evaluate such evidence to inform their own practice' (HCPC, 2017).

13.3.2 Law, social policy and ethical professional practice

When you are asked to write an assignment in health and social care, one of your learning outcomes for many of your assignments will be to discuss law and social policy. This is to demonstrate that you understand the law around your practice and that you will be practising safely. You will not need to know every law and policy, but you will need to know some key ones. These laws will help protect not only the vulnerable people we support but also ourselves as professional practitioners.

As health and social care practitioners we may find ourselves increasingly using policy and law to support our practice. This is not a bad thing to do, but it can be scary if you have never studied law before. The best way to think about policy and law is that it is there to help you make decisions with people and sometimes for them.

For example, one of the most common laws we now use is the Mental Capacity Act (Department of Health, 2005) because it helps us to help people to make decisions safely regardless of age or health status. Most laws also have a code of practice which is much easier to read than the statute itself and can help you to apply the law to practice much better. They are also usually free to download online. The five principles of the Mental

Capacity Act are designed to help you remember most of the law and to apply it ethically and professionally at all times.

THE FIVE PRINCIPLES OF THE MENTAL CAPACITY ACT (DOH, 2005) APPLIED TO PROFESSIONAL PRACTICE

Principle 1 – The person must be assumed to have capacity

Sometimes we are too quick to judge people without taking reasonable steps to find out if they can make a decision and that they have the capacity to do so; this principle reminds us of this.

Principle 2 – We must not treat people as unable to make decisions until we have tried to help them to do this

As health and social care professionals we need to be able to demonstrate that we have made reasonable attempts to help people understand information so that they can make a decision. For example, *not* when they are in pain or hungry.

Principle 3 – If people make an unwise decision, it is still a decision

Most of us will make unwise decisions at some stage in our life, but this does not mean that we do not have the capacity to make wise decisions. As health and social care professionals we will need to make sure that people understand that they have made an unwise decision and not punish them for it, for example, by withdrawing our services. (Neglect was first defined in this Act as a punishable offence.)

Principle 4 – Anything that we do to people must be in the person's best interests

Our interventions with people should remain focused upon their person-centred needs and not on the needs of other people or other services. This reminds us that we have to stay person-centred and not push people into existing services.

Principle 5 – A person's rights and freedom should be least restricted by whatever we do

If we do need to make decisions we should always limit the restrictions so that people can maintain their individual rights and freedom. This Act allowed health and social care practitioners to make decisions on behalf of people who may be too ill to make those decisions themselves, but those decisions should always be evidence-based and person-centred.

Using your professional codes and laws in your assignments and your applications for employment will help you to demonstrate your employability skills to your tutors and future employers. This in turn will help them to provide good character references for you and for your professional registration. Remember to reference the relevant code of practice, law or policy in your work to demonstrate your knowledge base and to avoid plagiarism.

13.4 Developing lifelong learning skills as a professional

When we become professional practitioners, or even before then, we are constantly developing individual awareness around our values, knowledge and actions, as suggested in the opening quote to this chapter. This process is also known as reflective practice, which is discussed in more detail in *Chapter 9*. Reflective practice can help us as professionals to demonstrate that we are constantly updating our knowledge. This applies not just when we are in training for a certain profession but also as a lifelong learning skill. This is known in the professional world as continuous professional development or CPD.

In professional practice and from the discussion above it becomes clear that a lot is expected of people in professional employment (Robertson *et al.*, 2016). We are not only expected to know a lot about what our jobs entail, but we are also required to demonstrate this in practice. In modern employment terms this means outcomes or outputs, which in general means our employers want to see what they are getting for their money.

Employers effectively buy our knowledge and time so they, like any other customer, want to buy good-quality services. In many professional jobs we are often asked to attend a Professional Development Review (PDR) to show our employers or managers how we are developing and to discuss what we might need to develop further. Our employer also needs to match our development to the development of the organisation. It is therefore important to be both assertive and reflective upon what our individual needs are and how they might fit with the organisation's needs. For example, you might like to learn to play the guitar, but your employer is not likely to pay for you to learn how to play the guitar if the organisation does not require guitar players. More importantly, as a skilled professional you will need to consider what skills and knowledge you will need to develop your career in the next 5, 10 or 20 years.

ACTIVITY 13.5: DEVELOPING A CAREER PATHWAY USING LIFELONG LEARNING SKILLS

Try using your lifelong learning skills to reflect upon where you would like to be at certain stages in your career and think about what skills and knowledge you might need to get there. Some examples are provided below.

Stages in my career	Level of development	Skills and knowledge needed
5 years' time	e.g. Manager	
10 years' time	e.g. Lecturer	
15 years' time		
20 years' time		

You may have already begun to notice that planning for your future automatically requires you to be more assertive and resilient. It also helps you to feel more in control of your own professional development as you plan how your career might turn out. There are no guarantees that it will turn out this way, but by using and developing lifelong learning skills early in your professional career you will feel more able to cope with the heavy demands that will be placed on you (Winbolt, 2016).

When preparing for a Professional Development Review (PDR), it is worth taking some time to reflect upon what you need to develop your career. These are also useful considerations for when you attend job interviews, where you might be asked at the end of the interview if you have any questions.

Some questions for you to ask at your interview:
Will I have study time? This is very important for you to develop your professional career, as we have already discussed above that you will need to keep learning and reflecting throughout your career to maintain your professional registration.
Will I have supervision? As a student you will have had lots of supervision from your tutors in education and from your mentors in practice. You may not have noticed this as supervision, but there is clear guidance provided by your professional bodies and by your university on how you should be supervised.
Will I be able to develop my career in this area of practice? This is linked to your employability skills as well as your lifelong learning skills because you will need to know how you can develop your knowledge further.
How do practitioners develop as a team in this area of practice? This is a good way to find out what developmental opportunities there are and how the whole team develops together.

Preparing for interview can be daunting, but if you think of it as a presentation, as suggested in *Chapter 11*, you will already be familiar with your own strengths and weaknesses in this area. You can then work on them a bit more to give a resilient and well-presented interview.

13.5 **Conclusion**

As Oxtoby (2016) suggests, we should always bear in mind what effect our professional practice has on others and therefore we need to be constantly reflecting upon how we can do this and keep our knowledge and skills up to date at the same time. Many professional organisations take professional development very seriously as they are aware that it can improve the quality of the service that they provide. Furthermore, in the light of many serious allegations against health and social care organisations, professional development is a huge part of risk management and quality improvement in practice. As professionals in health and social care we all have a duty to be providing the best possible care that we can.

Four key points to take away from *Chapter 13*:
- ☑ Professional practice can influence how others behave.
- ☑ Professional development is very important for good-quality care.
- ☑ Professional development is part of quality improvement.
- ☑ Professional development also includes risk management.

Quiz

1. How can I develop my resilience at work?
   a. Develop my skills
   b. Ask someone to help me
   c. Ignore my own needs

2. What does CPD stand for?
   a. Common Professional Development
   b. Continuous Professional Development
   c. Compressed Professional Development

3. What does PDR stand for?
   a. Public Development Review
   b. Personal Development Review
   c. Professional Development Review

4. What does the Hippocratic Oath mean?
   a. First help others
   b. First help yourself
   c. First do no harm

REFERENCES

Department of Health (2005) *Mental Capacity Act*. HMSO.

General Social Care Council (2011) *Professional Boundaries: guidance for social workers*. HMSO.

Health and Care Professions Council (2017) *Standards of Proficiency – social workers in England*. Health and Care Professions Council.

Heaslip, V. and Lindsay, B. (2019) *Research and Evidence-Based Practice: for nursing, health and social care students*. Lantern Publishing.

Jones, L. and Bennett, C.L. (2018) *Leadership: for nursing, health and social care students*. Lantern Publishing.

Nursing and Midwifery Council (2018a) *The Code: professional standards of practice and behaviour for nurses, midwives and nursing associates*. NMC.

Nursing and Midwifery Council (2018b) *Future Nurse: standards of proficiency for registered nurses*. NMC.

Oxtoby, K. (2016) Is the Hippocratic oath still relevant to practising doctors today? *BMJ Careers*, 2016, 355.

Robertson, H.D., Elliot, A.M. and Matherson, C. (2016) Resilience of primary healthcare professionals. A systematic review. *British Journal of General Practice*, 66(647), 423–33.

Winbolt, B. (2016) *9 Ways to Improve your Resilience at Work*. Online blog. Available at: www.barrywinbolt.com/resilience-at-work (accessed 9 September 2019).

Chapter 14
Lifelong learning skills: future-proof your learning

Peggy Murphy and Craig Morley

LEARNING OUTCOMES

When you have completed this chapter you should be able to:

14.1 Understand the importance of lifelong learning

14.2 Identify approaches to improve resilience in lifelong learning

14.3 Identify the professional requirements for lifelong learning linked to health and social care employability

14.4 Take advantage of opportunities for learning by fostering a growth mindset and developing your reflective practice

14.5 Future-proof lifelong learning through a love of learning about health and social care.

14.1 What is lifelong learning?

In this chapter we will be looking at how you can develop your lifelong learning (LLL) skills throughout your career and how this can start on the very first day of your studies. Often LLL is thought of as being organised and up-to-date in your knowledge, but it is much more than that. If you consider how long you will have to work and develop your skills in your chosen career, you will realise that LLL skills are something that is personal to you so that you can reach your career goals.

LLL has a range of definitions, including the following:

1. The continued learning of new skills and completion of qualifications (Department for Education and Skills, 2003)
2. A naturally occurring, universal process (Loads, 2007)
3. A means to empower people and encourage engagement with wide-ranging issues (European Commission, 2001)
4. An individual's duty and responsibility (Reeves *et al.*, 2002).

Regardless of the specific definition you decide upon, LLL is essential in meeting the challenges of the twenty-first century (Fryer, 1997). LLL affects both your professional and personal development. As a healthcare practitioner, LLL is an integral part of your day-to-day work. A career in health and social care means that there are new people to meet with different demands and a constant stream of new knowledge on how best to support people's needs. In order to cope with the constant challenges of the career you will need to be involved in LLL. This is not a passive process; it is an active process that requires your full participation. Activities that promote LLL can be both formal and informal. This can include:

- Training workshops
- Courses
- FE or HE qualifications
- Learning from others
- Reflection
- Sharing ideas, thoughts and best practice.

Learning can take place in university, in work or anywhere else and every interaction you have with others provides a learning opportunity.

14.2 Where does resilience fit into LLL?

Many different characteristics have been identified in successful lifelong learners. From a health and social care perspective the most relevant are (list adapted from: Mason-Whitehead and Mason, 2008; Nevison *et al.*, 2017):

- Resilience during learning challenges
- Self-directed learning strategies
- Self-reliance in working practices
- Being proactive and reactive to changing demands and expectations
- Having a love of learning.

14.2.1 Resilience during learning challenges

Building resilience, or developing a grittier approach to overcoming obstacles to learning, has been the focus of Duckworth's (2012) work. Duckworth found that a person's attitude towards learning challenges matters more than their innate ability or intelligence quotient, when predicting their likelihood of success.

14.2.2 Self-directed learning strategies

Independent learning is central to academic success at university and in career progression. According to the theory of andragogy, adult learners learn best when they direct their own learning (Knowles, 1973). This involves moving away from dependency on tutors or lecturers to become more self-directed. Taking responsibility for your own lifelong learning needs and ambitions creates feelings of empowerment and that you are in control of your own learning and career progression.

14.2.3 Self-reliance in working practices

Although you will more than likely be working as part of a team as a health and social care practitioner there will be elements of that work that you are completely and individually accountable for. Part of LLL in your career is to monitor your own progress towards becoming more reliant upon your own evaluation of your work, especially in specific areas.

14.2.4 Being proactive and reactive to changing demands and expectations

There are few careers that demand staff continually adapt to change more than health and social care. One way to gain some control in an ever-changing climate is to take charge of your learning and find direction for your own continuous professional development rather than simply reacting to change. Effective lifelong learners are better prepared to react and adapt to changes as and when they occur; therefore, they are more able to maintain high performance levels.

14.2.5 Having a love of learning

Skills you will learn at university that will enable you to be an effective lifelong learner:
- Evidence-based practice
- Reflection
- Critical evaluation.

In your assignments at university your work will often be judged by criteria like these. They are not merely abstract academic ideas, but are the underpinning elements of your success as an effective practitioner throughout your career.

14.3 Employability and lifelong learning skills

One way to protect yourself and sustain a demanding lifelong career is to recognise your humanity in the process of continuous development. If you can learn to feel OK about not feeling OK this can help you to move through the experiential stages of becoming an expert. Benner (1984) described these phases as moving from novice to an expert. This movement is not a linear process, and as you progress you may well return to being a novice from the dizzy heights of being an expert. Benner (1984) identified the stages in skill acquisition in particular that nurses pass through as novice, advanced beginner, competent, proficient and, lastly, expert (*Figure 14.1*).

Throughout your career you are likely to move from one 'comfort zone' into another. It is often this transitional phase that is the most anxiety-provoking, as challenging ourselves to develop can be scary. None of us really know what our full potential is, and there is always a risk of failure. This is when maintaining a growth mindset helps. If we continuously view 'failure' as a method to learn then failure becomes a lot less frightening. Embarking on a career in health and social care demands that we continuously develop ourselves as practitioners. Therefore, until we have challenged ourselves over a long period of time and moved from one level of proficiency to another, we can never really know what our

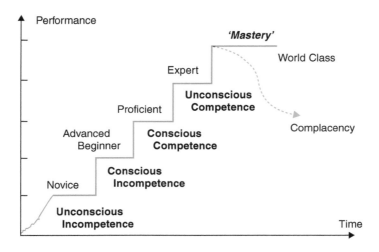

Figure 14.1 *The trajectory of novice to expert (Benner, 1984).*

full capacity to learn is. The road towards realising your full potential can be like a game of snakes and ladders and is rarely a straightforward path.

At the beginning of your career you are likely to feel very self-conscious as a new starter. It can appear that everyone else knows what they are doing. When you compare yourself against others you can find yourself wanting. Just remember that everyone had to start somewhere and nobody starts a career knowing everything. Every health and social care practitioner that has gone before you will have passed through various stages in their career. When you first start you do not realise what you do not know; in other words, you are unconsciously incompetent. As you pass through the stages you become acutely aware of how much you need to learn. This occurs through exposure to new experiences and learning from those experience. Eventually, you will reach a stage of unconscious competence (*Figure 14.2*). An example of this would be someone who is so skilled in breaking bad news to patients and families that they do not even remember what actions they took until they are questioned about them after the event, usually by a student.

14.4 Future-proofing learning to maintain professional standards

There is a professional requirement that health and social care practitioners keep abreast of new knowledge in order to inform their work and keep that practice 'current'. Embarking on a profession in health and social care involves being presented with many challenges and these can be viewed as learning opportunities if you maintain a growth mindset throughout your career. (See *Chapter 8* for more detail on the concept of the growth mindset.)

Many people choose this area of work because no two days are ever the same. Even when you have encountered a situation in health and social care work before, it is unlikely that two events will ever be the same. The nature of health and social care work requires you to work with communities, individuals, their families and carers alongside colleagues

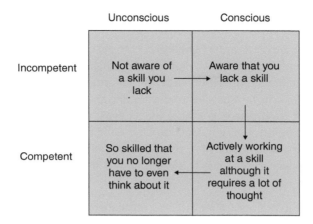

Figure 14.2 *Model demonstrating the stages from unconscious incompetence through to unconscious competence. The 'Four Stages for Learning Any New Skill' was developed at the Gordon Training International by Noel Burch in the 1970s.*

in a health and social care team. The people you work with may come from different backgrounds and cultures. Maintaining your curiosity about other humans and how they live will provide you with rich opportunities for learning and increase your cultural competence.

Health and social care work also takes place in an ever-changing landscape of new policy. There is an expectation that you will remain an evidence-based practitioner throughout your career; that you will be able to use current research to offer more effective ways to improve the lives of the people in your care. There are a number of ways to do this, but it may be important to consider how you will sustain your curiosity about the subject of your career for a lifetime. Maintaining your interest in health and social care and the people that you care for and work with throughout a whole career can be challenging. It helps if you have a natural inquisitiveness about people.

Fostering an effective approach to lifelong learning involves learning with and from others. There are formal learning opportunities that you can engage with, such as attending conferences and postgraduate courses. You may decide to develop your skills in research and engage in creating new knowledge about your field for future generations. Likewise, you can use job and performance appraisals to guide your personal and professional developmental requirements.

HELPFUL HINT

There are different approaches available to develop yourself within your daily practice. One way to maintain a focus on your personal and professional development and encourage LLL is to incorporate reflective practice into your daily work. You can do this by maintaining your own reflective journal. Reflective practice is an effective way to continuously assess your progress in order to develop your skills for life. Adopting this approach enables you to perceive every aspect of your career in health and social care as an opportunity to learn, develop and improve.

14.5 Future-proofing learning to maintain professional registration

Once you have embarked on a career in health and social care, it is likely your profession will be governed by a professional body. For example, the Nursing and Midwifery Council (NMC) state that to maintain registration with the NMC nurses and midwives must show they have engaged in a constant process of developing themselves professionally. The NMC require nurses to revalidate every three years; revalidation involves providing evidence of how lifelong learning impacts upon their ability to practise safely throughout their careers. Each nurse and midwife has to reflect on their practice, stay up to date and record their CPD. One way they can do this is by maintaining a portfolio of evidence (see *Chapter 12*).

The Health and Care Professions Council (HCPC) regulate many other professions in this field including occupational therapists, paramedics, physiotherapists, social workers and, in England, speech and language therapists. In order to maintain registration with the HCPC, registrants have to demonstrate that they have participated in regular CPD. Both the NMC and HCPC advise practitioners to keep records about how they have engaged in learning activities as a portfolio of evidence. They also advocate that practitioners consider ways that engaging in CPD improves practice and benefits service users. In order to ensure that registrants participate with CPD, the HCPC audit a random sample of each profession at every renewal.

 IMPROVING RESILIENCE, LIFELONG LEARNING AND EMPLOYABILITY

Maintaining your curiosity and developing your lifelong learning skills will help you in maintaining your professional registration.

ACTIVITY 14.1

Investigate the requirements and procedures for maintaining registration with the professional body responsible for your chosen field of practice.

14.6 Combining reflective practice with a growth mindset

Chapter 9 explored the concept of reflective practice. Adopting these principles enables you to contemplate the noteworthy occasions in your career and consider what you have learned from the process of looking back. One way to start becoming a reflective practitioner is to write a diary to log your thoughts and feelings, particularly around any elements of the job that have impacted upon you. If you do this you need to maintain the confidentiality of any person that you write about, so it is useful to consider any identifiable characteristics such as name and age and change them to ensure people's right to privacy.

Reflective practice allows you to think about and assess your performance in work and this gives you feedback from your self-evaluation. *Chapter 8* discussed feedback and the importance of working with feedback to facilitate personal and professional development. One concept that was discussed was Dweck's (2006) notion of the importance of adopting a 'growth mindset' in order to continuously develop. Educationalists including Petty (2009) and Mortiboys (2012) recognise that feedback can help students to realise that success and failure are more in their control than they may at first realise. Once you learn how to utilise feedback so you can recognise the difference between actual performance and desired performance (and seek guidance on how you can make improvements to reduce the gap) you will become more motivated. One way to embrace lifelong learning and shift from a fixed to a growth mindset is to weave in working with feedback throughout your career.

There are a number of models of reflective practice that you can utilise (see *Chapter 9*) and *Chapter 8* mentions a simple three step-approach: ***Stop*** doing … ***Start*** doing … ***Continue*** doing … There are many issues you may choose to reflect upon, including anything from building sufficient confidence to answer the phone in a work situation to dealing with a medical emergency (and anything in between). There are lots of opportunities for learning if you look for them and sometimes they come from the least likely sources, such as a complaint. Once you take a situation you may have initially perceived as having a negative effect on your career and reflect upon what you can learn from it you can develop personally and professionally and also improve your own mental health.

ACTIVITY 14.2: JOB DESCRIPTION

Below is an example of a job description and person specification. If you were to apply for this, how qualified would you be right now? Read through the job description and person specification, and identify:

- Which skills/requirements you already have
- Which skills/requirements you will need to develop
- Which skills/requirements you are currently working on

Job description

This is a level 3 role for a frontline colleague who will be supporting people with sensory difficulties (primarily sight and hearing problems). You may also be required to support people with complex learning needs.

You could be supporting children, adults or older adults and possibly a range of all the age groups.

The settings you will work in include:
Residential
Day activities
The Fibauld College

As a member of our team you will enable people to:
Have control over their lives
Decrease isolation
Maximise opportunities for people with sensory difficulties to fully participate in their communities.

Key responsibilities

Listen to and respond to people using communication they understand

Support people to learn new skills

Support people to maintain their health and well-being

Support people with personal care needs (if required)

Support people with their behaviour

Enable the people you support to influence the services and the way they are supported

Provide opportunities for people to make choices

Support people to run their own homes

Support people to keep in contact with family and friends

Keep all records up to date

Take part in supervision and attend meetings

Keep up to date with our policies and practices

Keep a safe and healthy environment for you, your colleagues and the people you support.

Person specification

Education and training	
Essential criteria	**Desirable criteria**
Has BSc in Health and Social Care or is willing to work towards one	An understanding of Deafblind Manual and Block Alphabet, to either have British Sign Language Level 1 or working towards it
Willing to complete Sense Communicator Guide training within a specified timescale	BSL Level two
	BSc in Health and Social Care or equivalent
Achievements and experience	
Essential criteria	**Desirable criteria**
Recent experience of working with people with sensory impairment, dual sensory impairment or people using a range of communication methods	Experience of working with/socialising with deaf/deafblind people/community
Experience of successfully mentoring and guiding colleagues	
	Experience of supporting people with behaviour that can challenge
Experience of planning care and keeping records related to people being supported	Experience of evidence-based practice
Experience of handling money and accounting for expenditure	Experience of handling money that belongs to other people

Experience of facilitating a person-centred review/individual learning plan	
Experience of working with acquired deafblind adults	
Skills and abilities	
Essential criteria	**Desirable criteria**
An ability to communicate effectively both in written and non-written format and in formal and informal settings	
An understanding of both congenital and acquired deafblindness and its implications	
Ability to work on own initiative and use good judgement, particularly when working in isolation	
The ability to build effective working relationships with others (e.g. colleagues, professional bodies and other significant people)	
Ability to keep appropriate and accurate records on the service	
Ability to support clients with mobility problems (e.g. assisting with walking, guiding or working with a person who is a wheelchair user)	
An ability to accompany/participate in leisure activities of the person's choice, for example collecting benefits, gym, swimming, accessing banks, attending groups, pubs, shopping, rallies, day trips, etc.	
To be able to travel from one place to another during working hours supporting the person(s)	
Ability to creatively solve problems using a person-centred approach	
Number and language skills in order to support individuals with their daily activities	
Ability to work in harmony with others on team activities	

After completing this activity, look for job descriptions and specifications for jobs that you are interested in. Identify which of these skills experiences you currently have and which you do not. Those you do not have will help you to plan your own professional development.

ACTIVITY 14.3: CAREER PLANNING

Thinking about your career progression and what you want to achieve in the short, medium and long term is an important step in planning your own professional development. Knowing where you want to go, and what you need to learn or achieve to get there, allows you to map out your own LLL.
One-year plan …
Five-year plan …
Ten-year plan …

HELPFUL HINT

It may also be worth thinking about the legacy that you wish to leave behind. People come into health and social care to make a difference; what 'difference' do you want to make? It may seem strange for you to contemplate this at the start of your career, but when we work to a deadline we can be more focused and effective. It may be helpful to think right from the start about how you would like to be remembered in your chosen field so you keep on track and remember throughout your career exactly what you are aiming for.

14.7 Conclusion

Developing lifelong learning skills is an important part of professional development if you intend to work and develop your career in health and social care. In a fast-changing environment of education and practice it is important not to feel too overwhelmed by the demands that this might make on you and to develop your resilience so that you can cope with these changing demands. In education, professional programmes of study are also changing to try and develop practitioners who can cope with the pace of change in health and social care practice, policy and law. If we accept that the future is going to be constantly changing we must prepare ourselves and our colleagues with the resilience and lifelong learning skills that will ensure we can manage these changes. In maintaining these skills we can be confident that our employability skills will also develop so that we can be part of developing and growing a rewarding and very valuable career.

SUMMARY

Four key points to take away from *Chapter 14*:
- ☑ Lifelong learning is very important in helping you develop your resilience and employability.
- ☑ Lifelong learning enables you to maintain and develop your study skills.
- ☑ Lifelong learning empowers you to plan your future career.
- ☑ Lifelong learning enables you to provide good-quality health and social care.

Quiz

1. What do we mean by lifelong learning?

2. Why is lifelong learning important in health and social care?

3. What are the five characteristics of effective lifelong learning?

REFERENCES

Benner, P. (1984) *From Novice to Expert: excellence and power in clinical nursing practice.* Addison-Wesley.

Department for Education and Skills (2003) *21st Century Skills: realising our potential*. DfEs.

Duckworth, A. (2012) *Grit*. Scribner.

Dweck, C.S. (2006) *Mindset: changing the way you think to fulfil your potential*. Random House.

European Commission (2001) *Communication from the Commission: making a European area of lifelong learning a reality*. European Commission.

Fryer, B. (1997) *Learning for the 21st Century*. Department of Education and Employment.

Knowles, M. (1973) *The Adult Learner: a neglected species*. American Society for Training and Development, Madison, WI. Full text available at: https://files.eric. ed.gov/fulltext/ED084368.pdf (accessed 9 September 2019)

Loads, D. (2007) Effective learning advisers' perception of their role in lifelong learning. *Teaching in Higher Education*, 12(2), 235–45.

Mason-Whitehead, E. and Mason, T. (2008) *Study Skills for Nurses* (2nd edition). Sage.

Mortiboys, A. (2012) *Teaching with Emotional Intelligence* (2nd edition). Routledge.

Nevison, C., Drewery, D., Pretti, J. and Cormier, L. (2017) Using learning environments to create meaningful work for co-op students. *Higher Education Research and Development*, 36, 807–22.

Petty, G. (2009) *Teaching Today: a practical guide* (4th edition). Nelson Thornes.

Reeves, F., Harrison, R., Edwards, R., Lore, A. and Cartwright, M. (2002) *E845 Supporting Lifelong Learning: study guide*. Open University.

FURTHER READING (FOR LIFELONG LEARNING)

Candy, P.C., Crebert, G. and O'Leary, J. (1994) *Developing Lifelong Learners through Undergraduate Education*. National Board of Employment, Education and Training Commissioned Report. Australian Government Publishing Service.

Forde-Johnston, C. (2018) *How to Thrive as a Newly Qualified Nurse*. Lantern Publishing.

Health and Care Professions Council www.hcpc-uk.org/aboutus

Knapper, C. and Cropley, A.J. (2000) *Lifelong Learning in Higher Education*. Psychology Press.

Nursing and Midwifery Council (2018) *The Code: professional standards of practice and behaviour for nurses, midwives and nursing associates*. Nursing and Midwifery Council. www.nmc.org.uk/standards/code/read-the-code-online

Answers to quizzes

Chapter 1

1. a
2. b
3. c
4. a
5. c

Chapter 2

1. b
2. a
3. c
4. a

Chapter 3

1. All
2. PubMed, Google Scholar, Google Books
3. a, b, c, e
4. a, c, d
5. b
6. a, b, c

Chapter 4

1. Grey, research, reports
2. What do I want to know and how will I limit my search?
3. What do I want to look at and what do I want to leave out?
4. Critically analysing the literature
5. Making sense of the literature

Chapter 5

1. Analysing and criticising information in order to apply a logical and informed approach to problem-solving.

2. Slowing down the thinking process, deep consideration, debating options, evaluating options for their strengths and weaknesses, comparing with additional literature.
3. Answer: 3
   - Critical reading
   - Identifying the premise
   - Scepticism
   - Constructing arguments,
   - Integrating the literature
   - Reflection.

4. Answer: 4
   - Critical thinking enhances resilience so that students have enhanced coping abilities when faced with stressful situations.
   - Critical thinking enhances interpersonal confidence to challenge working practice and question in many non-work situations.
   - Critical thinking is a lifelong transferable skill.
   - Critical thinking enhances understanding of academic work.
   - Critical thinking reduces the opportunity to make mistakes due to thinking being slowed down and more deliberate.
   - Critical thinking improves the quality of healthcare as practitioners are more know-ledgeable about the options that exist and they can debate which of the options are more suited for individuals to produce person-centred, safe care.

Chapter 6

1. d
2. c
3. a
4. d

Chapter 7

1. ISSN number
2. Publication details
3. Check your answer against the guidance provided in your university's referencing guide

Chapter 8

1. Feedback highlights the parts of work that were done well; it suggests what parts need improving; it offers information to accelerate learning and can be the start of a dialogue between lecturer and student
2. Accessing feedback from a number of sources is a professional requirement and helps students consider how they need to utilise a partnership approach to lifelong learning
3. Feed-forward applies to the process where feedback can be utilised to inform current work – an example would be submitting a draft of an assessment to get comments that help guide before a final submission

4. Becoming proactive about accessing feedback helps you to have a sense of control over it, recognising that feedback helps you develop promotes a growth mindset
5. Specific, Measurable, Achievable, Realistic and Timely
6. Read it and make an appointment to see your tutor to discuss it. Recognise any patterns in the areas you need to develop, access support services in the areas you require (study skills, library, tutors)
7. This means that you need to ask the question 'so what?', e.g. so what does this mean when demonstrating an inclusive approach to healthcare to the people who access the service?
8. This usually means that you have written a large section without stating where your ideas are from, or that you have written an emphatic statement, e.g. 'Nurses need to be good listeners', without stating where this information is from

Chapter 9

1. Kolb
2. Reflective writing
3. Perceptual acuity
4. Reflection in action
5. Reflection on action

Chapter 10

1. (a) an identity (in a workplace often identified by a name); (b) a shared goal; (c) members with interdependent roles
2. Forming, Storming, Norming, Performing
3. Adjourning
4. Practitioners work to their distinct professional roles in a multidisciplinary team, whereas in an interdisciplinary team practitioners work collaboratively.
5. In a 'pseudo' team, there is little interaction and objectives are unclear or unknown. In a 'real' team, there is frequent interaction and objectives are jointly agreed.

Chapter 11

1. Preparation, Planning and Practice
2. Gather the evidence you need for the presentation
3. Practise your presentation well before you deliver it
4. Become more self-aware of your skills and how you can improve them

Chapter 12

1. a
2. c
3. a
4. a

Chapter 13

1. a
2. b
3. c
4. c

Chapter 14

1. The continued learning of new skills and completion of qualifications; a naturally occurring, universal process, a means to empower people and encourage engagement with wide-ranging issues; an individual's duty and responsibility
2. There is a professional requirement that health and social care practitioners keep abreast of new knowledge in order to inform their work and keep that practice 'current'. Maintaining your curiosity about other humans and how they live will provide you with rich opportunities for learning and increasing your cultural competence.
3. Resilience during learning challenges; self-directed learning strategies; self-reliance in working practices; being proactive and reactive to changing demands and expectations; having a love of learning.

Index